OFFICIAL Instant Pot BOOK

The "I LOVE MY INSTANT POT®" ANTI-INFLAMMATORY DIET Recipe Book

From *Orange Ginger Salmon* to *Apple Crisp*, 175 Easy and Delicious Recipes That Reduce Inflammation

Maryea Flaherty of HappyHealthyMama.com
Author of *Anti-Inflammatory Drinks for Health*

Adams Media

New York London Toronto Sydney New Delhi

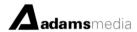

Adams Media
An Imprint of Simon & Schuster, Inc.
57 Littlefield Street
Avon, Massachusetts 02322

First Adams Media trade paperback edition October 2019

ADAMS MEDIA and colophon are trademarks of Simon & Schuster.

For information about special discounts for bulk purchases, please contact Simon & Schuster Special Sales at 1-866-506-1949 or business@simonandschuster.com.

The Simon & Schuster Speakers Bureau can bring authors to your live event. For more information or to book an event contact the Simon & Schuster Speakers Bureau at 1-866-248-3049 or visit our website at www.simonspeakers.com.

Interior design by Colleen Cunningham
Interior layout by Julia Jacintho
Photographs by James Stefiuk

Manufactured in the United States of America

10 9 8 7 6 5 4 3 2

Library of Congress Cataloging-in-Publication Data
Names: Flaherty, Maryea, author.
Title: The "I love my instant pot®" anti-inflammatory diet recipe book / Maryea Flaherty of HappyHealthyMama.com, author of Anti-inflammatory drinks for health
Description: Avon, Massachusetts: Adams Media, 2019.
Series: "I love my" series.
Includes index.
Identifiers: LCCN 2019023101 | ISBN 9781507210994 (pb) | ISBN 9781507211007 (ebook)
Subjects: LCSH: Pressure cooking. | One-dish meals. | Quick and easy cooking. | Cooking.
Classification: LCC TX840.P7 F55 2019 | DDC 641.5/87--dc23
LC record available at https://lccn.loc.gov/2019023101

ISBN 978-1-5072-1099-4
ISBN 978-1-5072-1100-7 (ebook)

Many of the designations used by manufacturers and sellers to distinguish their products are claimed as trademarks. Where those designations appear in this book and Simon & Schuster, Inc., was aware of a trademark claim, the designations have been printed with initial capital letters.

INSTANT POT® and associated logos are owned by Instant Brands Inc. and are used under license.

The information in this book should not be used for diagnosing or treating any health problem. Not all diet and exercise plans suit everyone. You should always consult a trained medical professional before starting a diet, taking any form of medication, or embarking on any fitness or weight-training program. The author and publisher disclaim any liability arising directly or indirectly from the use of this book.

Always follow safety and commonsense cooking protocols while using kitchen utensils, operating ovens and stoves, and handling uncooked food. If children are assisting in the preparation of any recipe, they should always be supervised by an adult.

Contents

Introduction

The anti-inflammatory diet seems to be everywhere today, but it's no fad diet. First of all, eating an anti-inflammatory diet just means eating real, whole, and unprocessed foods to promote a healthy inflammatory response in your body. Some of the most significant benefits to reducing your body's inflammation are decreasing your risk for conditions such as chronic body aches, persistent indigestion, and diseases such as fibromyalgia, heart disease, and cancer.

So, what exactly *is* inflammation and why do you want to avoid it? If you've ever had a cold, sprained your ankle, or scraped your knee, you've experienced inflammation. It is your body's natural, and necessary, response to outside stressors on your body such as injury or infection. Normally, once your body has the stressor under control the response turns off. However, when the inflammation response does not stop working and continues to function long after the original need, it can lead to damaging chronic inflammation in your body.

The good news is that you can help promote a healthy inflammatory response in your body *and* control and reduce chronic inflammation through healthy diet and lifestyle choices. Nature is filled with foods that contain powerful, inflammation-fighting nutrients. If you fill your plate with foods like brightly colored fruits and vegetables, herbs and spices, and healthy fats every day, you'll be on your way to promoting a healthy inflammatory response in your body.

In addition to eating anti-inflammatory foods, you'll also want to avoid or limit foods that can cause a harmful inflammatory response. Foods that are known to cause inflammation include refined carbohydrates found in foods like crackers, cakes, and bagels; foods containing gluten; dairy foods containing casein; foods with added sugars; and foods with trans fats, such as fried foods.

And that's where your Instant Pot® comes in. Cooking with an Instant Pot® is a life-changing experience, especially when you are trying to eat whole, healthy foods to fight inflammation. This multifunction cooking tool allows you to sauté, brown, steam, and warm your food. It cooks soups, eggs, and even cakes! And the high-pressure cooking and steaming ability of an Instant Pot® does wonders to steaks, pork shoulders, and chicken. With the touch of a button you'll be able to cook cuts of meat that would normally take hours upon hours in just minutes. In addition, the Instant Pot® actually cooks food at a lower temperature, but it does it more efficiently than other methods because the pressure denies steam to release. This cooking method also seals in essential vitamins and minerals, making it the ideal tool for your anti-inflammatory diet recipes.

Whether you've just bought your Instant Pot® or have been using one for years and just need some inspiration, this book is for you. Inside you'll find 175 delicious anti-inflammation recipes ranging from Orange Cinnamon Oatmeal Muffins (see recipe in Chapter 2) and Turkey Chili (see recipe in Chapter 3) to Asian Noodle Bowls (see recipe in Chapter 7) and Lemon Dill Salmon (see recipe in Chapter 8). You'll also find decadent desserts like Blueberry Crisp and Banana Chocolate Chip Bundt Cake (see recipes in Chapter 10). The more you cook, the more you'll realize how versatile the Instant Pot® really is, whether you're making a hearty breakfast, an amazing main course, or a delicious dessert. So plug in your Instant Pot® and get ready to enjoy some amazing, delicious, and quick anti-inflammation meals.

Cooking with an Instant Pot®

If you're excited to jump into the world of Instant Pot® cooking but aren't sure where or how to start, this chapter is for you. Here is where you will learn what all those buttons on your Instant Pot® mean, what they do, and when to use them. You'll find out how to release the pressure from your Instant Pot®, how to keep it clean, and which accessories you'll want to help you get the most from your user experience.

Even though this chapter is packed full of useful information, it's still important for you to start with your owner's manual. That manual is the first step to being a successful Instant Pot® user and having success with the recipes in this book. It will walk you through the basic functions of your pot as well as teach you how to do an initial test run with water. This is an important step in understanding how the Instant Pot® works, decreasing any anxiety you might have about using it, and giving it a good steam cleaning before you make your first recipe.

Function Buttons

When you look at the Instant Pot® you may become overwhelmed with all the buttons. Which one should you use? It's actually easy once you take a moment to read about the function of each button, and you'll learn that several are set with preprogrammed cooking times. You will likely use the Manual or Pressure Cook button the most frequently as it gives you the most control, but there will be times when you'll want to use the specialty buttons as well. Keep in mind that every button option on the Instant Pot® is programmed with a 10-second delay, meaning the cooking time will start 10 seconds after you hit the button.

Let's take a look at all of the different function buttons.

Manual/Pressure Cook Button

Depending on the model of the Instant Pot®, there is a button labeled either Manual or Pressure Cook. For most people, this is the most-used button on the Instant Pot®. The default pressure is set to high, however you can change the pressure from high to low by pressing the Pressure button. Then use the Plus and Minus buttons to adjust the pressurized cooking time that is correct for the food you are cooking.

Sauté Button

This button heats the inner pot and allows your Instant Pot® to act as a skillet for sautéing vegetables or browning meat prior to adding the remaining ingredients of a recipe. In addition, it can also be used for simmering sauces. There are three temperature settings that you can access using the Adjust button. The Normal setting is for sautéing, the Less setting is for simmering, and the More setting is for searing meat. The lid is kept open when using the sauté function.

Soup Button

This button is used to cook soups and broths at high pressure for a default of 30 minutes. The Adjust button allows you to change the cooking time to 20 or 40 minutes.

Porridge Button

This button is used to cook porridge at a high pressure for a default of 20 minutes. The Adjust button allows you to change the cooking time to 15 or 40 minutes.

Poultry Button

This is the button you'll use to cook chicken and turkey at high pressure for a default of 15 minutes. The Adjust button allows you to change the cooking time to 20 or 45 minutes.

Meat/Stew Button

This is the button you'll use if you're cooking red meat or stew meats, and it defaults to high pressure for 35 minutes. Using the Adjust button allows you to change the cooking time to 25 or 40 minutes.

Bean/Chili Button

This button is used to cook fried beans and chili at high pressure for a default of 30 minutes. The Adjust button allows you to change the cooking time to 25 or 40 minutes.

Rice Button

This button is used to cook white rice such as jasmine or basmati at low pressure. The Instant Pot® will automatically set the default cooking time by sensing the amount of water and rice in the cooking vessel.

Multigrain Button

This button is used to cooked grains such as wild rice or barley at high pressure for a default of 40 minutes. The Adjust button allows you to change the cooking time to 20 or 60 minutes.

Steam Button

This button is excellent for steaming vegetables and seafood using your steamer basket. It steams for a default of 10 minutes. The Adjust button allows you to change the cooking time to 3 or 15 minutes. Quick-release the steam immediately after the timer beeps so as to not overcook the food.

Slow Cook Button

This button allows the Instant Pot® to cook like a slow cooker. It defaults to a 4-hour cook time. The Adjust button allows you to change the temperature to Less, Normal, or More, which correspond to a slow cooker's Low, Normal, or High. The Plus and Minus buttons allow you to adjust the cooking time.

Keep Warm/Cancel Button

When the Instant Pot® is being programmed or in operation, pressing this button cancels the operation and returns it to a standby state. When the Instant Pot® is in the standby state, pressing this button again activates the Keep Warm function.

Automatic Keep Warm Function

After the cooking time is up in the Instant Pot®, the pot automatically switches over to the Keep Warm function and will keep your food warm for up to 10 hours. This is perfect for large cuts of meat as well as for soups, stews, and chili, allowing the flavors to be enhanced with time for an even better taste. The first digit on the LED display will show an L to indicate that the Instant Pot® is in the Keep Warm cycle, and the clock will count up from 0 seconds to 10 hours.

Timer Button

This button allows you to delay the start of cooking up to 24 hours. After you select a cooking program and make any time adjustments press the Timer button and use the Plus or Minus keys to enter the delayed minutes. You can press the Keep Warm/Cancel button to cancel the timed delay. The Timer function doesn't work with Sauté, Yogurt, and Keep Warm functions.

How Does Food Cook in 0 Minutes?

If you are confused about how some recipes call for 0 minutes to cook, it's not a typo. Certain foods like quicker-cooking vegetables and seafood that require only minimal steaming to cook are set at 0 minutes cooking time. These foods can actually be cooked in the time that it takes the Instant Pot® to achieve pressure.

Locking and Pressure-Release Methods

Other than the Sauté function, where the lid should be off, and the Slow Cook or Keep Warm functions, where the lid can be on or off, most of the cooking you'll do in the Instant Pot® will be under pressure, and that means you must know how to lock the lid before pressurized cooking and also how to safely release the pressure after cooking.

Once all of your ingredients are in the inner pot, lock the lid by putting it on the Instant Pot® with the triangle mark aligned with the Unlocked mark on the rim of the Instant Pot®. Then turn the lid 30 degrees clockwise until the triangle mark is aligned with the Locked mark on the rim. Turn the pointed end of the pressure release handle on top of the lid to the Sealing position. After your cooking program has ended or you've pressed the Keep Warm/Cancel button to end the cooking, there are two ways you can release the pressure.

Natural Release Method

To naturally release the pressure, simply wait until the Instant Pot® has cooled sufficiently for all the pressure to be released and the float valve drops. This typically takes about 10–15 minutes. You can either unplug the Instant Pot® while the pressure releases naturally or let pressure release while it is still on the Keep Warm function.

Quick-Release Method

The quick-release method ends the cooking process and helps unlock the lid for immediate serving. To quickly release the pressure of the Instant Pot®, make sure you are wearing oven mitts, then turn the pressure release handle to the Venting position to let out steam until float valve drops. This is generally not recommended for starchy foods or recipes with a lot of liquid, such as soup, to avoid splattering that could occur. Be prepared, because the noise and geyser effect of releasing steam during the quick-release method can be quite surprising the first time.

Pot-in-Pot Accessories

Pot-in-pot cooking is when you place another cooking dish inside the Instant Pot® for a particular recipe. The Instant Pot® comes with an inner pot and steam rack; however, there are many other accessories that will allow you to expand what you can do with your new cooking tool. Let's take a look at the different options.

Although the accessories listed here can help you branch out and make different recipes with the Instant Pot®, know that there are plenty of recipes you can make with just your inner pot or your inner pot and steam rack that came with your appliance. These are just handy extras to gather along the way as you expand what you like to cook in your Instant Pot®.

7" Springform Pan

A 7" springform pan is perfect for a number of desserts in the Instant Pot®. It is the right dimension to fit in the Instant Pot® and makes a dessert for four to six people.

7-Cup Glass Bowl

A 7-cup bowl fits perfectly in your Instant Pot® and works great for eggs, bread puddings, or dips that would normally burn on the bottom of the pot insert. The bowls

sits up on the inserted steam rack and the food inside is cooked with the steam and pressure of the pot.

5" and 6" Cake Pans

5" and 6" cake pans are excellent for making small cakes in the Instant Pot®. The Instant Pot® will make a cake that will serve 4–6 people, depending on serving size. It works perfectly for a family craving a small dessert but preferring no leftovers. These pans are also excellent for making breads and bars as traditional bread and square pans don't fit in the Instant Pot®.

Ramekins

These small baking dishes (typically 4 ounces) are the perfect vessels for individual dishes from breakfast to dessert.

Steamer Basket

A steamer basket helps create a raised shelf for steaming. You can shop around and find several variations, including metal or silicone steamer baskets. Some even have handles to make it easier to remove after the cooking process while the steamer is hot.

Silicone Baking Cupcake Liners

These liners are for so much more than cupcakes. They are perfect for mini turkey meatloaves, portable frittatas, muffins, and quick breads.

Accessory Removal

Cooking pot-in-pot is a great idea, but you must take care to remove the inserted cooking dish from the tight space. If you try to do this with just thick oven mitts, there's a good chance you'll tip the cooking vessel to the side and spill your cooked food. Here are some handy tools to prevent that from happening,

These tools will help you when you're using pot-in-pot cooking, but are not necessary if you are simply using the interior pot that comes with the appliance upon purchase. A spoon or slotted spoon will do the trick for most other meals.

Retriever Tongs

Retriever tongs are a helpful tool for removing hot pans from the Instant Pot®.

Mini Mitts

Small oven mitts are helpful when lifting pots out of an Instant Pot® after the cooking process. Silicone mitts that fit just over your fingers and thumbs work especially well.

Aluminum Foil Sling

This is a quick, inexpensive fix to the problem of lifting a heated dish out of the Instant Pot®. To create the sling, take a 10" × 10" square of aluminum foil and fold it back and forth until you have a 2" × 10" sling. Place this sling underneath the bowl or pan before cooking so that you can easily lift up the heated dish.

Cleaning Your Instant Pot®

When cleaning up after using your Instant Pot®, the first thing you should do is unplug it and let it cool down. Then you can break down the following parts to clean and inspect for any trapped food particles:

Inner Pot

This is the cooking vessel, and it's dishwasher safe; however, the high heat can cause discoloration on stainless steel. To avoid this, hand wash your inner pot.

Outer Heating Unit

Wipe the interior and exterior with a damp cloth. Never submerge this in water, as it's an electrical appliance.

Steam Rack

The steam rack is dishwasher safe or can be cleaned with soap and water.

Lid

The lid needs to be broken down into individual parts before washing. The sealing ring, the float valve, the pressure release handle, and the antiblock shield all need to be cleaned in different ways:

- **Sealing ring.** Once this ring is removed, check the integrity of the silicone. If it gets torn or cracked, it will not seal properly and may hinder the cooking process, in which case it should not be used. The sealing ring needs to be removed and washed each time because it has a tendency to hold odors when cooking. Vinegar and lemon juice are excellent for reducing odors. You can purchase additional rings for a nominal price. Many Instant Pot® owners choose to do so and use one for meats and their extra one for desserts and milder dishes.
- **Float valve.** The float valve is a safety feature that serves as a latch lock that prevents the lid from being opened during the cooking process. Check to ensure this valve can move easily and is not obstructed by any food particles.

- **Pressure-release handle.** This is the venting handle on top of the lid and it can be pulled out for cleaning. It is naturally loose because it needs to be able to move when necessary.
- **Antiblock shield.** The antiblock shield is the little silver "basket" underneath the lid. It is located directly below the vent. This shield can and should be removed and cleaned. It blocks any foods, especially starches, so they don't clog the vent.

What Is Inflammation?

The inflammatory response is completely normal and is the cornerstone of the body's healing response. It is simply the way the body supplies nourishment and enhanced immune activity to areas experiencing injury or infection.

Whenever you are exposed to an infectious agent or experience tissue injury or damage, your immune system mounts an inflammatory response. For example, when you cut your finger and it becomes red and swollen, inflammation goes to work, and it's a lifesaver. Blood flow increases to places that require healing. Pain intensifies as a signal that something is wrong within the body. And compounds such as eicosanoids (also known as *prostaglandins*, *prostacyclins*, *thromboxanes*, and *leukotrienes*) are released to attack unwelcome foreign invaders such as bacteria while tending to harmed tissue. Under normal circumstances, once the threat is under control, anti-inflammatory substances are released to turn off the immune response.

Sometimes, however, inflammation gets the upper hand and continues to operate chronically. This causes continual secretion of pro-inflammatory chemicals in the body. The chronic release and circulation of these chemicals results in an attack on healthy cells, blood vessels, and tissues.

Chronic inflammation generates a wide range of symptoms, including:

- Frequent body aches and pains
- Chronic stiffness
- Loss of joint function
- Recurrent swelling
- Persistent indigestion
- Regular bouts of diarrhea
- Unrelenting skin outbreaks

Over time, chronic inflammation acts like a slow but deadly poison, causing overzealous inflammatory chemicals to damage your body as you innocently go about your normal daily activities. Other diseases and conditions thought to be associated with chronic inflammation include, but are not limited to:

- Allergies
- Asthma
- Cancer
- Crohn's disease
- Fibromyalgia
- Inflammatory bowel disease (IBD)
- Heart disease
- Kidney failure
- Psoriasis
- Rheumatoid arthritis (RA)
- Stroke

Foods That Increase Inflammation

Research shows that one of the main culprits contributing to chronic inflammation is the food you eat. Certain foods have the ability to trigger inflammation in the body, and when you eat those foods daily, it causes chronic inflammation. It's just as important to stay away from inflammatory foods as it is to add anti-inflammatory foods to your diet.

Advanced Glycation End Products (AGEs)

Researchers have identified chemical reactions that occur in the body that lead to the production of pro-inflammatory substances called *advanced glycation end products* (AGEs). AGEs do not exist in nature but are produced during food processing. Regardless of their source, all AGEs have been shown to exacerbate inflammation. In a nutshell, the foods high in AGEs are highly processed, refined foods such as:

- Frankfurters, bacon, and powdered egg whites
- Fast foods such as French fries, hamburgers, and fried chicken
- Prepackaged foods that have been preserved, pasteurized, homogenized, or refined, such as white flour, cake mixes, processed cereals, dried milk, dried eggs, pasteurized milk, and canned or frozen precooked meals
- Cream cheese, butter, margarine, mayonnaise, and dried fruits

Trans Fats

Nothing could be more inflammation-promoting than trans fats. These fats lead to the synthesis of pro-inflammatory prostaglandins. Foods that tend to be high in trans fats include:

- Fried and deep-fried foods (these are usually cooked in hydrogenated shortening)

- Margarine and shortening
- Nondairy creamers
- Baked goods such as cakes, pie crusts, and cookies (especially those with frosting)
- Biscuits
- Doughnuts
- Crackers, chips, and other snack foods that contain the word *hydrogenated* in the ingredient list

Other Inflammatory Foods

- **Saturated fats.** Saturated fats are nonessential fats commonly found in meats, high-fat dairy products, and eggs. Although these foods provide important vitamins and minerals, saturated fats can promote inflammation, which is demonstrated by their ability to increase the fibrinogen and CRP inflammatory biomarkers in the blood.
- **Omega-6 fatty acids.** Although they are unsaturated and considered essential in small quantities, excessive intake of omega-6 fatty acids promotes inflammation, encourages blood clotting, and can cause cells in the body to proliferate uncontrollably. The modern diet is weighed down by omega-6 fatty acids because of overconsumption of meats and vegetable oils such as corn, safflower, soybean, and cottonseed that are commonly found in processed foods and fast foods.
- **Nightshades.** Although fruits and vegetables are extremely beneficial to your health, there are certain vegetables that are members of the nightshade family of plants that may exacerbate inflammation in some people, including: potatoes, tomatoes, eggplants, ground cherries, and tomatillos.

Foods That Fight Inflammation

Thankfully, there are a myriad of foods that can help your body fight inflammation. In fact, the most powerful inflammation fighters can be found in the grocery store, not the pharmacy! Your best bet is to shop mostly the perimeter of the supermarket where you find fresh, unprocessed foods. Look for a wide variety of brightly colored fruits and vegetables, herbs and spices, and foods with healthy fats. Let's take a closer look at all the inflammation-fighting foods you should be filling your grocery cart up with!

Fruits and Vegetables

Fruits and vegetables are major storehouses of phytochemicals and antioxidants, both of which have anti-inflammatory powers. Phytochemicals are chemicals found in plants, and although they are not essential for life, their benefits are far-reaching, such as helping to reduce the risk of cancer, heart disease, and diabetes. Plants rely on phytochemicals for their own protection and survival. These potent chemicals help plants resist the attacks of bacteria and fungi, the potential havoc brought on by free radicals, and the constant exposure to ultraviolet light from the sun. Fortunately, when you consume plants, the plants' chemicals infuse into your body's tissues and provide ammunition against disease.

Omega-3 Fatty Acids

Omega-3 fatty acids have an anti-inflammatory effect in the body. These fatty acids are converted into hormone-like substances called *eicosanoids*. The two most potent omega-3 eicosanoids are eicosapentaenoic acid (EPA) and docosahexaenoic acid (DHA). EPA and DHA have the overall effect of dilating blood vessels, minimizing blood clotting, and reducing inflammation. Foods high in omega-3s include:

- Fatty fish such as albacore tuna, anchovies, Atlantic herring, halibut, lake trout, mackerel, sardines, stripped sea bass, and wild salmon
- Flaxseeds and flaxseed oils
- Walnuts
- Soybeans
- Tofu

Probiotics

All humans have millions and millions of naturally occurring bacteria in their bodies. Normally, bacteria get a bad rap, but the right types of bacteria, specifically lactobacilli and bifidobacteria, can keep you healthy and even prevent disease. More specifically, these bacteria support the immune system, keeping it strong and better able to fend off disease and illness. They also have anti-inflammatory effects in the gut that can be helpful in treating constipation, diarrhea, inflammatory bowel disease, and irritable bowel syndrome.

You can help good bacteria flourish by consuming foods that contain high concentrations of healthy probiotics (the term *probiotics* means "for life") such as *Lactobacillus acidophilus*. Fermented milk products such as yogurt, kefir, and some soy-based beverages will increase the probiotic bacteria within your body. Look on the label for the "live and active cultures" statement to ensure that you are increasing your consumption of probiotics.

Lean Protein

Lean meats, white-meat poultry, and eggs will give you clean protein without excessive amounts of pro-inflammatory fats. Cold-water fish offer plenty of quality protein with a kick of anti-inflammatory omega-3 fatty acids.

Vegetable proteins, such as soy foods, beans, lentils, whole grains, seeds, and nuts, will further reduce the presence of pro-inflammatory agents in the body while giving you a blast of phytochemicals and antioxidants.

Garlic

Garlic is a potent anti-inflammatory power food. It contains chemicals that crush the inflammation-promoting substances in the body. As a result, regular garlic consumption can help minimize the side effects of asthma and reduce the pain and inflammation associated with osteoarthritis and rheumatoid arthritis.

Curcumin

Curcumin is a substance found in the yellow curry spice, turmeric. Curcumin is touted as having antioxidant powers, anti-inflammatory qualities, and possibly even anticancer effects. Preliminary findings from animal studies suggest that curcumin may actually possess anti-inflammatory and anticancer properties, but currently very little research exists that evaluates the actual effects of curcumin supplementation on disease risk in humans.

Ginger

Ginger is a tropical plant and a relative of turmeric. Certain constituents of ginger, referred to as *gingerols*, are touted to inhibit numerous biochemicals that promote inflammation, especially in cases of osteoarthritis and rheumatoid arthritis. Fresh ginger adds a light spiciness and mellow sweetness to dishes and is a wonderful spice to incorporate into stir-fries and dipping sauces.

Let's Get Cooking

So, now that you know what foods you should eat, which you should avoid, and how to use all the safety features, buttons, and parts on your Instant Pot®, you are ready to start your cooking adventure! Get ready to dive into healthy, anti-inflammatory recipes with what will quickly become your new favorite cooking appliance!

2

Breakfast

Whether you're looking for quick and easy weekday breakfast ideas, or you hope to find the perfect recipe to serve at your next brunch, this chapter has you covered. The Instant Pot® is the perfect tool to help you prepare a nutritious breakfast in no time at all.

Eating a healthy, anti-inflammatory breakfast doesn't have to be difficult, complicated, bland, or boring. You'll find a wide variety of nutritious breakfast recipes in this chapter and will be amazed at how delicious this way of eating can be.

Looking for warm and cozy? Check out the Banana Walnut Steel Cut Oats. Fancy a more savory breakfast? Try the Egg Casserole with Kale. Maybe you want to try something different? You'll love exploring new textures with the Blueberry Vanilla Quinoa Porridge. Sometimes all you need to start your day on the right foot is a big bowl of vegetables. Try the Vegetable Breakfast Bowls.

There is something for every member of the family in this chapter of breakfast recipes. Don't let breakfast become a chore. Use this chapter to help you start your day with food that both fuels you and satisfies you.

Egg Casserole with Kale

Kale is one of the most nutrient-dense and powerful anti-inflammatory foods on the planet. When paired with eggs in this mouthwatering egg casserole, it's easy to love it. Garlic, rosemary, and thyme give this frittata an amazing flavor that you'll love. This is also a perfect recipe for meal prep. Make it once and heat it up for breakfast for the next few days.

- **Hands-On Time: 10 minutes**
- **Cook Time: 17 minutes**

Serves 6

1 tablespoon avocado oil
1 small yellow onion, peeled and chopped
5 large kale leaves, tough stems removed and finely chopped
1 clove garlic, diced
2 tablespoons lemon juice
½ teaspoon salt, divided
9 large eggs
2 tablespoons water
1½ teaspoons dried rosemary
1 teaspoon dried oregano
¼ teaspoon black pepper
½ cup nutritional yeast

BENEFITS OF NUTRITIONAL YEAST
Nutritional yeast is your secret weapon for creating cheese-like flavor without adding dairy to your dishes. Not only does it have great flavor, it is also an excellent source of B vitamins.

1 Add the oil to the pot, press the Sauté button and heat oil for 1 minute.

2 Add the onion and sauté 2 minutes until just softened.

3 Add the kale, garlic, lemon juice, and ¼ teaspoon salt. Stir and allow to cook 2 minutes more. Press the Cancel button.

4 Meanwhile, in a medium bowl, whisk together the eggs, water, rosemary, oregano, ¼ teaspoon salt, pepper, and nutritional yeast.

5 Add the onion and kale mixture to the egg mixture and stir to combine.

6 Rinse the inner pot, add 2 cups water, and place a steam rack inside.

7 Spray a 7" springform pan with cooking spray. Transfer the egg mixture to the springform pan.

8 Place the pan on the steam rack and secure the lid. Press the Manual or Pressure Cook button and adjust time to 12 minutes.

9 When the timer beeps, quick-release pressure until float valve drops and then unlock lid.

10 Remove the pan from pot and allow to cool 5 minutes before slicing and serving.

CALORIES: 157 | **FAT:** 9g | **PROTEIN:** 13g | **SODIUM:** 311mg
FIBER: 2g | **CARBOHYDRATES:** 5g | **SUGAR:** 1g

Raspberry Steel Cut Oatmeal Bars

Steel cut oats are the perfect base for these wholesome and hearty breakfast bars. Made with delicious raspberries, you'll love the tart flavor mixed with the nutty flavor of the steel cut oats. Steel cut oats also provide a chewy texture and you can eat these bars with your hands or a fork!

- **Hands-On Time: 5 minutes**
- **Cook Time: 15 minutes**

Serves 6

3 cups steel cut oats

3 large eggs

2 cups unsweetened vanilla almond milk

⅓ cup erythritol

1 teaspoon pure vanilla extract

¼ teaspoon salt

1 cup frozen raspberries

1 In a medium bowl, mix together all ingredients except the raspberries. Once the ingredients are well combined, fold in the raspberries.

2 Spray a 6" cake pan with cooking oil. Transfer the oat mixture to the pan and cover the pan with aluminum foil.

3 Pour 1 cup water into the Instant Pot® and place the steam rack inside. Place the pan with the oat mixture on top of the rack. Secure the lid.

4 Press the Manual or Pressure Cook button and adjust the time to 15 minutes.

5 When the timer beeps, quick-release pressure until float valve drops and then unlock lid.

6 Carefully remove the pan from the inner pot and remove the foil. Allow to cool completely before cutting into bars and serving.

CALORIES: 399 | **FAT**: 9g | **PROTEIN**: 18g | **SODIUM**: 192mg
FIBER: 12g | **CARBOHYDRATES**: 72g | **SUGAR**: 1g

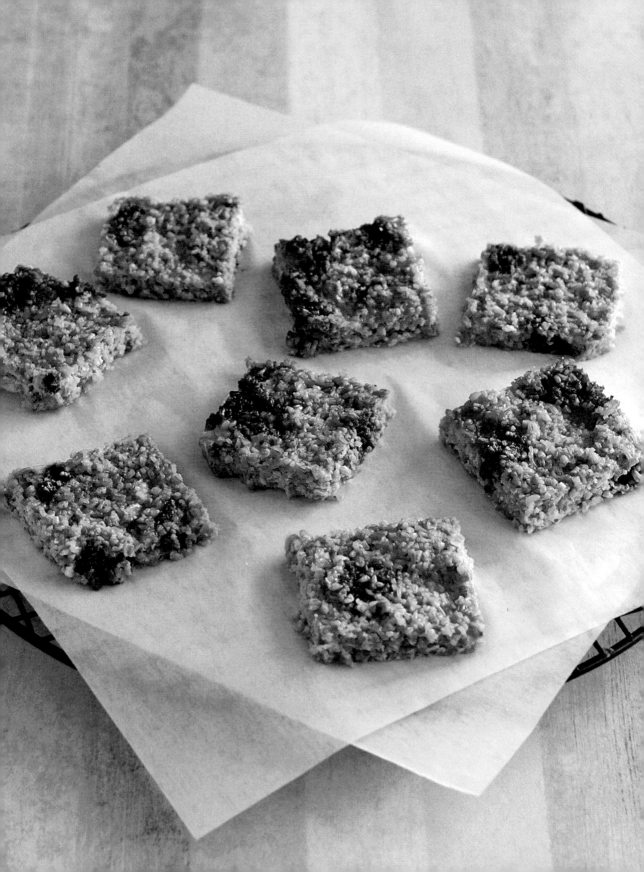

Blueberry Vanilla Quinoa Porridge

There's nothing more comforting on chilly mornings than a warm bowl of porridge. This porridge is made with quinoa, which is an ancient seed and is one of the only plant-based sources that contains a complete protein. The Instant Pot® is perfect for making this porridge quickly, making it ideal for busy mornings.

- **Hands-On Time: 2 minutes**
- **Cook Time: 1 minute**

Serves 6

1½ cups dry quinoa
3 cups water
1 cup frozen wild blueberries
½ teaspoon pure stevia powder
1 teaspoon pure vanilla extract

BITTER QUINOA?

If you've ever had quinoa that tasted bitter, it's probably because you didn't rinse it well enough. Quinoa is coated with a substance called saponin, and it has a naturally bitter taste. Rinsing your quinoa well will wash away the saponin and the bitter taste.

1 Using a fine-mesh strainer, rinse the quinoa very well until the water runs clear.

2 Add the quinoa, water, blueberries, stevia, and vanilla to the inner pot. Stir to combine. Secure the lid.

3 Press the Manual or Pressure Cook button and adjust the time to 1 minute.

4 When the timer beeps, quick-release pressure until float valve drops and then unlock lid.

5 Allow the quinoa to cool slightly before spooning into bowls to serve.

CALORIES: 181 | **FAT**: 3g | **PROTEIN**: 6g | **SODIUM**: 9mg
FIBER: 5g | **CARBOHYDRATES**: 33g | **SUGAR**: 3g

Buckwheat Ginger Granola

Traditional granola gets a new twist by adding hearty and nutritious buckwheat groats. Despite its name, buckwheat isn't wheat and contains no gluten. It's a highly digestible grain with antioxidants that can help control inflammation. It also has a nutty flavor that is perfect for your breakfast bowl. Paired with fresh ginger this is the most unique bowl of granola you'll ever eat.

- **Hands-On Time: 10 minutes**
- **Cook Time: 10 minutes**

Serves 8

1½ cups raw buckwheat groats

1½ cups old fashioned rolled oats

⅓ cup walnuts, coarsely chopped

⅓ cup unsweetened shredded coconut

¼ cup coconut oil, melted

1" piece fresh ginger, peeled and grated

3 tablespoons date syrup

1 teaspoon ground cinnamon

¼ teaspoon salt

THE POWER OF GINGER
Ginger is one of the most potent anti-inflammatory foods on the planet. The main compound in ginger responsible for this action is gingerol. Consuming ginger after intense physical exercise can help reduce muscle pain.

1 In a medium bowl, mix together the buckwheat groats, oats, walnuts, and shredded coconut until well combined. Add the coconut oil, ginger, date syrup, cinnamon, and salt and stir to combine.

2 Transfer this mixture to a 6" cake pan.

3 Pour 1 cup water into the inner pot and place a steam rack inside. Place the pan on the rack. Secure the lid.

4 Press the Manual or Pressure Cook button and adjust the time to 10 minutes.

5 When the timer beeps, quick-release pressure until float valve drops and then unlock lid.

6 Spread the granola onto a large sheet pan and allow it to cool, undisturbed, for 1 hour. It will crisp as it cools.

CALORIES: 311 | **FAT**: 13g | **PROTEIN**: 7g | **SODIUM**: 78mg
FIBER: 6g | **CARBOHYDRATES**: 42g | **SUGAR**: 6g

Orange Cinnamon Oatmeal Muffins

Orange and cinnamon are the perfect combination in these oatmeal muffins. You never have to worry about dry, crumbly muffins when you use your Instant Pot®. They turn out moist every time, and the pressure cooking locks in the flavor. Rolled oats are the base of these muffins, and the recipe yields six muffins.

- **Hands-On Time: 7 minutes**
- **Cook Time: 15 minutes**

Serves 6

3 cups old fashioned rolled oats
1 teaspoon baking powder
¼ teaspoon salt
1 teaspoon ground cinnamon
¼ cup unsweetened vanilla almond milk
¼ cup fresh orange juice
3⅓ cups mashed bananas
1 large egg
¼ cup erythritol

1 In a medium bowl, mix all of the ingredients together, stirring until well combined.

2 Place six silicone muffin cups inside of a 6" cake pan. Spoon the oatmeal mixture into the muffin cups. Cover the pan with aluminum foil.

3 Pour 1 cup water into the inner pot and place the steam rack inside. Place the cake pan with the muffins on the rack. Secure the lid.

4 Press the Manual or Pressure Cook button and adjust the time to 15 minutes.

5 When the timer beeps, quick-release pressure until float valve drops and then unlock lid.

6 Carefully remove the pan from the inner pot and remove the foil from the top. Let the muffins cool 15 minutes before eating. They will become firmer as they cool.

CALORIES: 318 | FAT: 5g | PROTEIN: 10g | SODIUM: 198mg
FIBER: 9g | CARBOHYDRATES: 70g | SUGAR: 17g

Coconut Chocolate Oatmeal

No one will ever believe that this decadent breakfast is a nutrient-dense, anti-inflammatory way to start your day. Coconut milk gives it its creamy, rich texture, and cacao powder is rich in polyphenols that contribute to its anti-inflammatory properties.

- **Hands-On Time: 5 minutes**
- **Cook Time: 6 minutes**

Serves 4

1 cup steel cut oats

1 (13.25-ounce) can full-fat unsweetened coconut milk

2 cups water

½ cup cacao powder

½ cup erythritol

⅛ teaspoon sea salt

1 Place the oats, coconut milk, water, cacao powder, erythritol, and salt in the inner pot and stir to combine. Secure the lid.

2 Press the Manual or Pressure Cook button and adjust the time to 6 minutes.

3 When the timer beeps, quick-release pressure until float valve drops and then unlock lid.

4 Allow the oatmeal to cool slightly before spooning into bowls to serve.

CALORIES: 394 | FAT: 23g | PROTEIN: 11g | SODIUM: 60mg
FIBER: 7g | CARBOHYDRATES: 62g | SUGAR: 0g

Banana Date Porridge

Bananas and dates naturally sweeten this warm breakfast without the need for any added sweeteners.

- **Hands-On Time: 5 minutes**
- **Cook Time: 4 minutes**

Serves 4

1 cup buckwheat groats

1½ cups unsweetened vanilla almond milk

1 cup water

1 large banana, mashed

5 pitted dates, chopped

¾ teaspoon ground cinnamon

¾ teaspoon pure vanilla extract

1 Place the buckwheat groats, almond milk, water, banana, dates, cinnamon, and vanilla in the inner pot and stir. Secure the lid.

2 Press the Manual or Pressure Cook button and adjust the time to 4 minutes.

3 When the timer beeps, quick-release pressure until float valve drops and then unlock lid.

4 Allow the porridge to cool slightly before spooning into bowls to serve.

CALORIES: 211 | FAT: 2g | PROTEIN: 6g | SODIUM: 72mg
FIBER: 6g | CARBOHYDRATES: 46g | SUGAR: 10g

Blueberry Banana Baked Oatmeal

Baked oatmeal is a filling, nutritious, and comforting breakfast you can make quickly and easily in the Instant Pot®. Instead of waiting 40 minutes for your breakfast to bake, you'll have breakfast on the table in less than 20 minutes. Baked oatmeal is thicker than regular oatmeal, but still produces a creamy bowl of oats. Mashed bananas add to the delightful texture and give a flavor reminiscent of warm banana bread, and the blueberries add a boost of anti-inflammatory antioxidants!

- **Hands-On Time: 5 minutes**
- **Cook Time: 7 minutes**

Serves 6

3 cups old fashioned rolled oats
¼ teaspoon salt
2 large bananas, mashed (1 heaping cup)
2 large eggs, lightly beaten
⅓ cup xylitol

1 In a medium bowl, place the oats, salt, bananas, eggs, and xylitol and stir to combine well.

2 Lightly spray a 6" cake pan with cooking spray. Transfer the oat mixture to the pan.

3 Pour 1½ cups water into the inner pot. Place a steam rack in the inner pot and place the pan on the steam rack. Secure the lid.

4 Press the Manual or Pressure Cook button and adjust the time to 7 minutes.

5 When the timer beeps, quick-release pressure until float valve drops and then unlock lid.

6 Allow the oatmeal to cool 5 minutes before serving.

CALORIES: 280 | FAT: 5g | PROTEIN: 10g | SODIUM: 120mg
FIBER: 6g | CARBOHYDRATES: 53g | SUGAR: 7g

Banana Walnut Steel Cut Oats

The Instant Pot® is the ideal tool for cooking steel cut oats—no more babysitting your pot on the stovetop. The oats cook perfectly in the pressure cooker with a creamy texture. This banana walnut version is sweetened naturally with just bananas and no added sugar. Spiked with cinnamon and vanilla, it has a lovely flavor, and both oats and walnuts have anti-inflammatory properties.

- **Hands-On Time: 2 minutes**
- **Cook Time: 4 minutes**

Serves 4

2 cups steel cut oats

2½ cups water

2½ cups unsweetened vanilla almond milk

3 medium bananas, thinly sliced

1½ teaspoons ground cinnamon

1 teaspoon pure vanilla extract

¼ teaspoon salt

4 tablespoons walnut pieces

1 Add the steel cut oats, water, almond milk, banana slices, cinnamon, vanilla, and salt to the Instant Pot® and stir to combine. Secure the lid.

2 Press the Manual or Pressure Cook button on the Instant Pot® and adjust the time to 4 minutes.

3 When the timer beeps, let pressure release naturally for 15 minutes, then quick-release any remaining pressure until float valve drops, then unlock lid.

4 Serve the oatmeal in a bowl topped with 1 tablespoon walnut pieces for each serving.

CALORIES: 491 | **FAT**: 13g | **PROTEIN**: 17g | **SODIUM**: 258mg
FIBER: 14g | **CARBOHYDRATES**: 81g | **SUGAR**: 11g

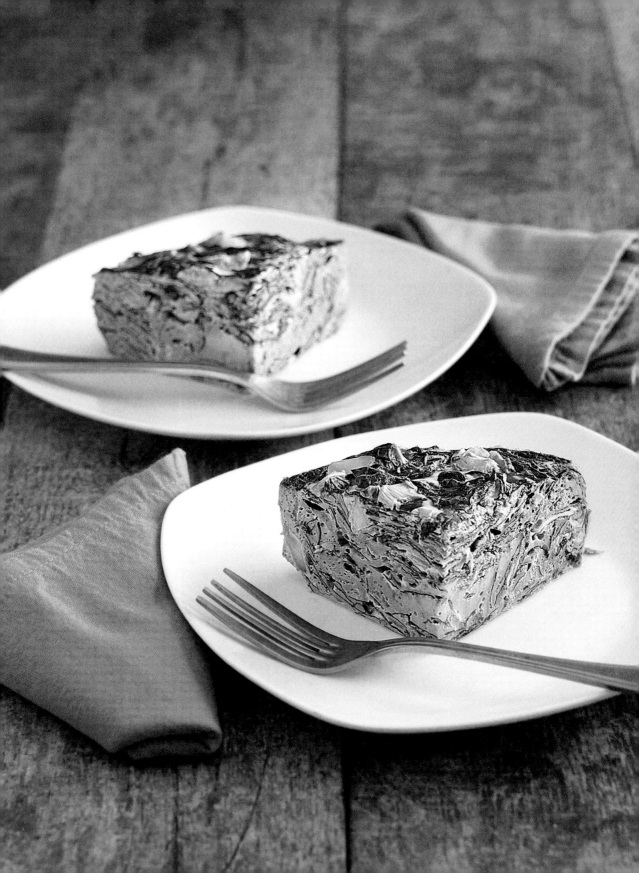

Spinach and Artichoke Egg Casserole

Spinach and artichoke pair so well together and also pack a nutritional punch. Step up your egg game with this Spinach and Artichoke Egg Casserole. With fresh chives and lemon, the flavors are bright in this satisfying breakfast that is ideal to serve a crowd with very little hands-on prep time.

- **Hands-On Time: 10 minutes**
- **Cook Time: 18 minutes**

Serves 8

12 large eggs
¼ cup water
4 cups baby spinach, roughly chopped
1 (14-ounce) can baby artichoke hearts, drained and roughly chopped
1 tablespoon chopped fresh chives
1 tablespoon fresh lemon juice
¾ teaspoon table salt
½ teaspoon black pepper
¼ teaspoon garlic salt

1 Spray a 6" round pan or 7-cup round glass bowl with cooking spray.

2 In a medium bowl, whisk together the eggs and water.

3 Stir in the spinach, artichokes, chives, lemon juice, table salt, pepper, and garlic salt.

4 Transfer the mixture to the prepared pan.

5 Place 2 cups water in the inner pot and place the steam rack inside. Place the pan on top of the steam rack. Secure the lid.

6 Press the Manual or Pressure Cook button and adjust the time to 18 minutes.

7 When the timer beeps, quick-release pressure until float valve drops and then unlock lid.

8 Remove egg casserole from pot and allow to cool 5 minutes before slicing and serving.

CALORIES: 122 | FAT: 7g | PROTEIN: 10g | SODIUM: 603mg
FIBER: 1g | CARBOHYDRATES: 3g | SUGAR: 1g

Coconut Almond Granola

All of the cereal lovers out there are going to love this Coconut Almond Granola. That's right; cereal can be healthy, and it's never been easier to make. If you've ever burned a pan of granola in your oven, you're going to be thankful you have an Instant Pot® for making perfect granola. This granola gets crunchier as it cools, so make sure you use the cooling time.

- **Hands-On Time: 5 minutes**
- **Cook Time: 7 minutes**

Serves 8

1½ cups old fashioned rolled oats
½ cup unsweetened shredded coconut
¼ cup monk fruit sweetener
⅛ teaspoon salt
¾ cup almond butter
¼ cup coconut oil

1 In a medium bowl, mix together the oats, coconut, sweetener, and salt. Add the almond butter and oil and mix until well combined.

2 Spray a 6" cake pan with nonstick cooking oil. Transfer the oat mixture to the pan.

3 Add 1 cup water to the inner pot of your Instant Pot®. Place the steam rack inside, and place the pan on top of the steam rack. Secure the lid.

4 Press the Manual or Pressure Cook button and adjust the time to 7 minutes.

5 When the timer beeps, quick-release pressure until float valve drops and then unlock lid.

6 Remove the pan from the inner pot and transfer the granola to a baking sheet to cool completely (at least 30 minutes) before serving.

CALORIES: 307 | FAT: 22g | PROTEIN: 8g | SODIUM: 37mg
FIBER: 5g | CARBOHYDRATES: 24g | SUGAR: 2g

Pumpkin Quinoa Porridge

Quinoa cooks to fluffy perfection in the Instant Pot®, and when you mix it with pumpkin purée it becomes a creamy porridge that is just sweet enough and bursting with flavors of cinnamon, clove, and nutmeg. All of these spices happen to have anti-inflammatory properties, but their warm, comforting flavors are what you'll remember about this special breakfast.

- **Hands-On Time: 2 minutes**
- **Cook Time: 1 minute**

Serves 4

¾ cup dry quinoa

2 cups water

¾ cup pumpkin purée

¼ cup monk fruit sweetener

1½ teaspoons pumpkin pie spice

1 teaspoon pure vanilla extract

¼ teaspoon salt

PUMPKIN IS FOR MORE THAN JUST PIE

While pumpkin pie is delicious, it's worth adding pumpkin to your diet in other ways as well. It's high in fiber and also has the powerful antioxidant beta-carotene.

1 Using a fine-mesh strainer, rinse the quinoa very well until the water runs clear.

2 Add the quinoa, water, pumpkin purée, sweetener, pumpkin pie spice, vanilla, and salt to the inner pot. Stir to combine. Secure the lid.

3 Press the Manual or Pressure Cook button and adjust the time to 1 minute.

4 When the timer beeps, quick-release pressure until float valve drops and then unlock lid.

5 Allow the quinoa to cool slightly before spooning into bowls to serve.

CALORIES: 141 | FAT: 2g | PROTEIN: 5g | SODIUM: 148mg
FIBER: 3g | CARBOHYDRATES: 37g | SUGAR: 2g

Meyer Lemon Poppy Seed Individual Baked Oatmeal Cups

Oatmeal cooks to creamy perfection with built-in portion control when you cook this breakfast in individual ramekins. Meyer lemons are naturally sweeter than regular lemons, and they lend that sweetness to these luscious breakfast treats. If you don't have Meyer lemons available, substitute regular lemons and use a teaspoon more erythritol.

- **Hands-On Time: 5 minutes**
- **Cook Time: 5 minutes**

Serves 4

2 cups old fashioned rolled oats
1 teaspoon baking powder
2 tablespoons erythritol
1 tablespoon poppy seeds
¼ teaspoon salt
1 large egg
Juice and zest from 1 Meyer lemon
1 cup unsweetened vanilla almond milk

1 Lightly grease four (8-ounce) ramekin dishes. Set aside.

2 In a medium bowl, mix together the oats, baking powder, erythritol, poppy seeds, and salt. Add the egg, juice and zest from the lemon, and the almond milk and stir to combine. Divide the oatmeal mixture into the four dishes.

3 Pour ½ cup water into the inner pot of the Instant Pot®. Place the steam rack inside the inner pot and place the ramekins on top of the rack. Secure the lid.

4 Press the Manual or Pressure Cook button and adjust the time to 5 minutes.

5 When the timer beeps, quick-release pressure until float valve drops and then unlock lid.

6 The ramekins will be hot when you open the lid, so be sure to use your mini oven mitts to lift them out of the Instant Pot® and let them cool before serving.

CALORIES: 229 | FAT: 6g | PROTEIN: 9g | SODIUM: 330mg
FIBER: 9g | CARBOHYDRATES: 40g | SUGAR: 1g

Apple Cinnamon Steel Cut Oats

Steel cut oats cook in a fraction of the time in your Instant Pot® compared to the stovetop, and when paired with apples and cinnamon, you've got a delicious, hearty, and healthy breakfast.

- **Hands-On Time: 10 minutes**
- **Cook Time: 4 minutes**

Serves 6

2 cups steel cut oats

3 cups unsweetened vanilla almond milk

3 cups water

3 small apples, peeled, cored, and cut into 1"-thick chunks

2 teaspoons ground cinnamon

¼ cup date syrup

¼ teaspoon salt

1 Add the steel cut oats, almond milk, water, apple chunks, cinnamon, date syrup, and salt to the Instant Pot® and stir to combine. Secure the lid.

2 Press the Manual or Pressure Cook button and adjust the time to 4 minutes.

3 When the timer beeps, let pressure release naturally for 15 minutes, then quick-release any remaining pressure until float valve drops, then unlock lid.

4 Serve warm.

CALORIES: 311 | **FAT**: 6g | **PROTEIN**: 10g | **SODIUM**: 193mg
FIBER: 8g | **CARBOHYDRATES**: 57g | **SUGAR**: 15g

Triple Berry Steel Cut Oats

Three different kinds of berries bring triple goodness to this creamy bowl of steel cut oats. Using frozen berries ensures they don't get too mushy with the pressure cooking.

- **Hands-On Time: 5 minutes**
- **Cook Time: 4 minutes**

Serves 6

2 cups steel cut oats

3 cups unsweetened almond milk

3 cups water

1 teaspoon pure vanilla extract

⅓ cup monk fruit sweetener

¼ teaspoon salt

1½ cups frozen berry blend with strawberries, blackberries, and raspberries

1 Add the steel cut oats, almond milk, water, vanilla, sweetener, and salt to the Instant Pot® and stir to combine. Place the frozen berries on top. Secure the lid.

2 Press the Manual or Pressure Cook button on the Instant Pot® and adjust the time to 4 minutes.

3 When the timer beeps, let pressure release naturally for 15 minutes, then quick-release any remaining pressure until float valve drops, then unlock lid. Serve warm.

CALORIES: 262 | **FAT**: 6g | **PROTEIN**: 10g | **SODIUM**: 187mg
FIBER: 9g | **CARBOHYDRATES**: 55g | **SUGAR**: 3g

Banana Pancake Bites

Pancake bites have the texture and flavor of pancakes, but in the form of a small muffin that you can eat with your hands! The silicone inserts that were designed for cooking egg muffins are perfect for these Banana Pancake Bites. Make sure you allow them to cool completely before trying to remove and they will come out without sticking. I recommend dipping your bites in pure maple syrup or spreading them with a little almond butter!

- **Hands-On Time: 10 minutes**
- **Cook Time: 6 minutes**

Serves 3

1¾ cups old fashioned rolled oats

3 small ripe bananas

3 large eggs

2 tablespoons erythritol

1 teaspoon ground cinnamon

1 teaspoon pure vanilla extract

1 teaspoon baking powder

PERFECT FINGER FOOD

If you have a toddler at home, these Banana Pancake Bites are the perfect shape for little fingers to pick up easily. They even work well for a snack on the go, so grab one before you head out with your toddler in the stroller!

1 Place the oats, bananas, eggs, erythritol, cinnamon, vanilla, and baking powder in a large, powerful blender and blend until very smooth, about 1 minute.

2 Pour the mixture into a silicone mold with seven wells. Place a paper towel on top and then top with aluminum foil. Tighten the edges to prevent extra moisture getting inside. Place the mold on top of your steam rack with handles.

3 Pour 1 cup water into the inner pot. Place the steam rack and mold inside. Secure the lid.

4 Press the Manual or Pressure Cook button and adjust the time to 6 minutes.

5 When the timer beeps, quick-release pressure until float valve drops and then unlock lid.

6 Pull the steam rack and mold out of the Instant Pot® and remove the aluminum foil and paper towel. Allow the pancake bites to cool completely, and then use a knife to pull the edges of the bites away from the mold. Press on the bottom of the mold and the pancake bites will pop right out.

CALORIES: 389 | **FAT**: 9g | **PROTEIN**: 16g | **SODIUM**: 234mg
FIBER: 9g | **CARBOHYDRATES**: 70g | **SUGAR**: 14g

Cinnamon Flaxseed Breakfast Loaf

Cinnamon and flaxseeds work together to bring you double anti-inflammatory powers in this satisfying breakfast loaf. There is nothing better than a warm slice of bread for breakfast, and this recipe does it without the usual refined flours and sugars. Even though it's made in a round pan, you can slice this loaf up just like regular bread.

- **Hands-On Time: 10 minutes**
- **Cook Time: 30 minutes**

Serves 6

½ cup ground golden flaxseed meal

½ cup almond flour

1 tablespoon ground cinnamon

2 teaspoons baking powder

½ teaspoon salt

⅔ cup xylitol

4 large eggs

½ cup coconut oil, melted and cooled

1 In a medium bowl, whisk together the flaxseed meal, flour, cinnamon, baking powder, salt, and xylitol.

2 In a separate medium bowl, whisk together the eggs and cooled coconut oil. Pour the wet ingredients into the dry ingredients and stir to combine.

3 Grease a 6" cake pan well and pour the mixture into the pan and cover with aluminum foil.

4 Pour 1½ cups water into the inner pot and place the steam rack with handles in the pot. Place the cake pan on top of the steam rack. Secure the lid.

5 Press the Manual or Pressure Cook button and adjust the time to 30 minutes.

6 When the timer beeps, quick-release pressure until float valve drops and then unlock lid. Carefully remove the pan from the Instant Pot® and allow the bread to cool completely before flipping the pan upside down and removing the loaf. Slice and serve.

CALORIES: 389 | **FAT**: 30g | **PROTEIN**: 9g | **SODIUM**: 407mg
FIBER: 6g | **CARBOHYDRATES**: 29g | **SUGAR**: 1g

Vegetable Breakfast Bowls

I can't think of a more nutritious way to start your day than with a bowl of vegetables. Turns out, it can be a totally satisfying breakfast, as well. This savory breakfast is full of nutrients that will fight inflammation and the flavor will leave you wondering when healthy food became so delicious.

- **Hands-On Time: 10 minutes**
- **Cook Time: 16 minutes**

Serves 2

2 tablespoons avocado oil

3 leeks, white and light green portion thinly sliced

8 ounces sliced baby bella mushrooms

½ teaspoon salt

¼ teaspoon black pepper

2 large carrots, peeled and sliced

5 kale leaves, tough stems removed and finely chopped

Juice from ½ medium lemon

1 Add the oil to the inner pot and turn on the Sauté button. Allow the oil to heat 2 minutes and then add the leeks, mushrooms, salt, and pepper. Sauté the leeks and mushrooms 10 minutes. Press the Cancel button.

2 Add the carrots, kale, and lemon juice and stir to combine. Secure the lid.

3 Press the Manual or Pressure Cook button and adjust the time to 4 minutes.

4 When the timer beeps, quick-release pressure until float valve drops and then unlock lid.

5 Serve immediately.

CALORIES: 270 | **FAT**: 14g | **PROTEIN**: 6g | **SODIUM**: 671mg
FIBER: 6g | **CARBOHYDRATES**: 33g | **SUGAR**: 11g

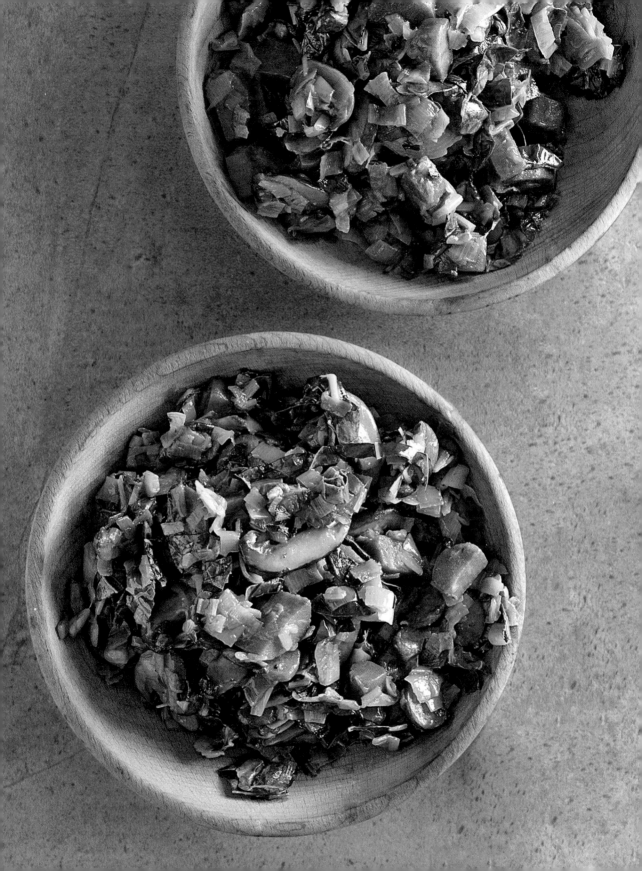

Root Vegetable Egg Casserole

Round up your root vegetables and make this cozy egg casserole. Fresh thyme complements the hearty vegetables perfectly and gives this egg casserole great flavor. The Instant Pot® speeds up the process as egg casseroles can take up to an hour in the oven, but don't forget to let it cool completely before slicing to give it time to set.

- **Hands-On Time: 10 minutes**
- **Cook Time: 29 minutes**

Serves 4

1 tablespoon avocado oil
1 small yellow onion, peeled and diced
1 small turnip, peeled and diced
1 medium parsnip, peeled and diced
2 small carrots, peeled and diced
1 teaspoon kosher salt
8 large eggs
1 tablespoon lemon juice
1 tablespoon fresh thyme leaves

1 Add the oil to the inner pot and press the Sauté button. Allow the oil to heat 1 minute and then add the onion, turnip, parsnip, carrots, and salt. Cook until the vegetables are softened, 10 minutes. Press the Cancel button.

2 In a medium bowl, whisk together the eggs and lemon juice. Add the thyme and vegetable mixture and stir to combine.

3 Spray the inside of a 7-cup glass bowl with cooking spray. Transfer the egg mixture to the bowl.

4 Add 1 cup water to the inner pot and place the steam rack inside. Place the bowl on top of the steam rack. Secure the lid.

5 Press the Manual or Pressure Cook button and adjust the time to 18 minutes.

6 When the timer beeps, quick-release pressure until float valve drops and then unlock lid.

7 Remove bowl from pot and allow to cool 5 minutes before slicing and serving.

CALORIES: 221 | **FAT**: 12g | **PROTEIN**: 14g | **SODIUM**: 754mg
FIBER: 3g | **CARBOHYDRATES**: 12g | **SUGAR**: 5g

Strawberries and Cream Quinoa Porridge

Strawberries and coconut milk pair together perfectly in this tasty quinoa porridge. Quinoa provides protein and fiber, and is also a filling breakfast choice. Coconut milk's fat content gives a creamy texture without dairy, and this is sweetened with just a touch of stevia powder.

- **Hands-On Time: 2 minutes**
- **Cook Time: 1 minute**

Serves 6

1½ cups dry quinoa

1½ cups water

1 (13.66-ounce) can unsweetened full-fat coconut milk

½ teaspoon pure stevia powder

1 teaspoon pure vanilla extract

1 cup sliced strawberries

⅓ cup unsweetened shredded coconut

1 Using a fine-mesh strainer, rinse the quinoa very well until the water runs clear.

2 Add the quinoa, water, coconut milk, stevia, and vanilla to the inner pot. Stir to combine. Secure the lid.

3 Press the Manual or Pressure Cook button and adjust the time to 1 minute.

4 When the timer beeps, quick-release pressure until float valve drops and then unlock lid.

5 Stir in strawberries. Allow the quinoa to cool slightly before spooning into bowls to serve. Top each bowl with a portion of the coconut.

CALORIES: 323 | **FAT**: 18g | **PROTEIN**: 8g | **SODIUM**: 10mg
FIBER: 4g | **CARBOHYDRATES**: 32g | **SUGAR**: 2g

Soft-Boiled Eggs with Asparagus

If you've never experienced soft-boiled eggs, you're in for a treat. When you break open the white, you'll find a runny yolk that acts as a sauce for the asparagus here. The Instant Pot® takes the guesswork out of soft-boiling your eggs and makes them perfectly cooked every time.

- **Hands-On Time: 2 minutes**
- **Cook Time: 3 minutes**

Serves 1

2 large eggs
5 large asparagus spears, woody ends removed

1 Place the whole eggs and asparagus into the steamer basket.

2 Pour 1 cup water into the inner pot and place the steam rack inside. Place the steamer basket with the eggs and asparagus on the rack. Secure the lid.

3 Press the Manual or Pressure Cook button and adjust the time to 3 minutes.

4 Prepare an ice bath by filling a large bowl with cold water and ice.

5 When the timer beeps, quick-release pressure until float valve drops and then unlock lid.

6 Carefully remove the steamer basket from the inner pot. Place the eggs into the ice bath until they have cooled enough to handle. Peel the eggs and serve with the asparagus.

CALORIES: 163 | **FAT**: 9g | **PROTEIN**: 15g | **SODIUM**: 144mg
FIBER: 2g | **CARBOHYDRATES**: 5g | **SUGAR**: 2g

3

Soups, Stews, and Chilis

Nothing beats the flavor of homemade soup, stews, and chilis—they just don't taste the same when they come from a can. The Instant Pot® allows you to get all of the outstanding flavor that homemade soups have but in a fraction of the time.

Soups make a healthy and easy one-pot dinner option, and the Instant Pot® helps you have it ready in less than an hour, and in many cases even 30 minutes! This is healthy eating at its easiest.

Homemade soups, stews, and chilis are also a convenient way to pack a variety of anti-inflammatory foods into one meal. The recipes in this chapter are filled with some of the most potent anti-inflammatory foods on the planet. You'll find delicious soups that include deeply pigmented vegetables and spices known to fight inflammation.

Once you master making homemade broth in your Instant Pot®, you'll be able to save money by using nutrient-dense homemade bone and vegetable broth in all of your soups, stews, and chilis.

There is a variety of vegetarian and vegan options in this chapter, along with some soups with chicken and turkey. All of these recipes are, of course, dairy- and gluten-free.

Chicken Bone Broth

Homemade bone broth is rich in nutrients and is known to be healing and restorative. Making your own bone broth can save you money and ensure it's full of all the wonderful benefits without any unwanted ingredients. Making your bone broth in the Instant Pot® eliminates the need to have a boiling pot on your stovetop for an entire day. This recipe gets the job done in just over 2 hours total!

- **Hands-On Time: 10 minutes**
- **Cook Time: 90 minutes**

Serves 8

Bones from a 3–4 pound chicken
8 cups water
2 large carrots, cut into chunks
2 large stalks celery, cut into chunks
1 large onion, peeled and cut into chunks
3 fresh rosemary sprigs
3 fresh thyme springs
2 tablespoons apple cider vinegar
1 teaspoon kosher salt

1 Put all of the ingredients in the Instant Pot® and allow it to sit 30 minutes.

2 Press the Manual or Pressure Cook button and adjust the time to 90 minutes.

3 When the timer beeps, let pressure release naturally until float valve drops and then unlock lid.

4 Strain the broth using a fine-mesh strainer and transfer into a storage container. The broth can be refrigerated three to five days or frozen up to six months.

CALORIES: 44 | FAT: 1g | PROTEIN: 7g | SODIUM: 312mg
FIBER: 0g | CARBOHYDRATES: 0g | SUGAR: 0g

HOW TO USE HOMEMADE BONE BROTH
Homemade bone broth can be used as is for an anti-inflammatory sipping beverage. It also makes the best base for many of the soup, stew, and chili recipes in this chapter.

Chicken Bone Broth with Ginger and Lemon

Chicken bone broth is already filled with nutrients, but add some fresh ginger and lemon and the health effects are compounded. This makes a great base for many soups, or simply use this as a healthy sipping broth.

- **Hands-On Time: 10 minutes**
- **Cook Time: 90 minutes**

Serves 8

Bones from a 3–4 pound chicken

8 cups water

2 large carrots, cut into chunks

2 large stalks celery, cut into chunks

1 large onion, peeled and cut into chunks

3 fresh rosemary sprigs

3 fresh thyme springs

2 tablespoons apple cider vinegar

1 teaspoon kosher salt

1½" piece fresh ginger, sliced (peeling not necessary)

1 large lemon, cut into fourths

1 Put all of the ingredients in the Instant Pot® and allow it to sit 30 minutes.

2 Press the Manual or Pressure Cook button and adjust the time to 90 minutes.

3 When the timer beeps, let pressure release naturally until float valve drops and then unlock lid.

4 Strain the broth using a fine-mesh strainer and transfer into a storage container. Can be refrigerated five days or frozen six months.

CALORIES: 44 | **FAT**: 1g | **PROTEIN**: 7g | **SODIUM**: 312mg
FIBER: 0g | **CARBOHYDRATES**: 0g | **SUGAR**: 0g

Vegetable Stock

Making your own vegetable stock could not be easier or quicker than when you use the Instant Pot®. Even better, you'll save money as well. Use this tasty stock in any soup that calls for a vegetable stock base. You can adjust the flavor of this broth based on your preferences. Play with the vegetables you use, get creative, and find your favorite combination using this base recipe as your guide. Vegetables need to be washed, but there is no need to peel.

- **Hands-On Time: 10 minutes**
- **Cook Time: 40 minutes**

Serves 8

2 large carrots
1 large onion, peeled and cut in half
2 large stalks celery
8 ounces white mushrooms
5 whole cloves garlic
2 cups parsley leaves
2 bay leaves
2 teaspoons whole black peppercorns
2 teaspoons kosher salt
10 cups water

1 Place all of the ingredients in the Instant Pot®. Secure the lid.

2 Press the Manual or Pressure Cook button and adjust the time to 40 minutes.

3 When the timer beeps, let pressure release naturally until float valve drops and then unlock lid.

4 Strain the broth using a fine-mesh strainer and transfer into a storage container. Can be refrigerated three to five days or frozen up to six months.

CALORIES: 9 | FAT: 0g | PROTEIN: 0g | SODIUM: 585mg
FIBER: 0g | CARBOHYDRATES: 2g | SUGAR: 1g

NO WASTE HERE
Vegetable scraps, like carrot peels and the ends of celery, can be used to make homemade vegetable stock. Save your scraps in a freezer-safe container and keep them in the freezer up to six months until you have enough to make a stock!

Chicken Vegetable Soup

They say chicken noodle soup is the perfect soup when you're sick, but it's a better idea to skip the noodles and add more vegetables! This Chicken Vegetable Soup tastes just like your favorite classic, but without the noodles that can contribute to inflammation.

- **Hands-On Time: 23 minutes**
- **Cook Time: 15 minutes**

Serves 8

2 tablespoons avocado oil

1 small yellow onion, peeled and chopped

2 large carrots, peeled and chopped

2 large stalks celery, ends removed and sliced

3 cloves garlic, minced

1 teaspoon dried thyme

1 teaspoon salt

8 cups chicken stock

3 boneless, skinless, frozen chicken breasts

1 Press the Sauté button and heat the oil in the inner pot 1 minute. Add the onion, carrots, and celery and sauté 8 minutes.

2 Add the garlic, thyme, and salt and sauté another 30 seconds. Press the Cancel button.

3 Add the stock and frozen chicken breasts to the pot. Secure the lid.

4 Press the Manual or Pressure Cook button and adjust the time to 6 minutes.

5 When the timer beeps, let pressure release naturally for 10 minutes, then quick-release any remaining pressure until float valve drops, then unlock lid.

6 Allow to cool slightly before ladling into bowls to serve.

CALORIES: 209 | **FAT**: 7g | **PROTEIN**: 21g | **SODIUM**: 687mg
FIBER: 1g | **CARBOHYDRATES**: 12g | **SUGAR**: 5g

Carrot Ginger Soup

Fresh ginger gives this soup a small bite and also packs a powerful anti-inflammatory punch. Ginger is one of the most potent anti-inflammatory spices you can use, and it pairs perfectly with carrot in this light and healthy soup. Serve this with a spring greens salad for a lunch you'll want to eat every week.

- **Hands-On Time: 20 minutes**
- **Cook Time: 21 minutes**

Serves 4

1 tablespoon avocado oil
1 large yellow onion, peeled and chopped
1 pound carrots, peeled and chopped
1 tablespoon fresh peeled and minced ginger
1½ teaspoons salt
3 cups vegetable broth

1 Press the Sauté button and add the oil to the inner pot, allowing it to heat 1 minute.

2 Add the onion, carrots, ginger, and salt and sauté 5 minutes. Press the Cancel button.

3 Add the broth and secure the lid. Press the Manual or Pressure Cook button and adjust the time to 15 minutes.

4 When the timer beeps, let pressure release naturally until float valve drops and then unlock lid.

5 Allow the soup to cool a few minutes, and then transfer to a large blender. Blend on high until smooth and then serve.

CALORIES: 99 | FAT: 4g | PROTEIN: 1g | SODIUM: 1,348mg
FIBER: 4g | CARBOHYDRATES: 16g | SUGAR: 7g

Tuscan White Bean Soup

This hearty white bean soup is perfect for chilly fall evenings! The flavor is spot on and it's easy to prepare. The dried beans cook right along with the rest of the soup, and much faster than if you used the stovetop. Red pepper flakes add just enough heat to make this soup interesting.

- **Hands-On Time: 10 minutes**
- **Cook Time: 22 minutes**

Serves 4

½ **pound dry white beans**

2 **tablespoons avocado oil**

1 **large yellow onion, peeled and diced**

2 **medium carrots, peeled and diced**

3 **medium stalks celery, ends removed and diced**

3 **cloves garlic, minced**

¾ **teaspoon kosher salt**

¼ **teaspoon ground white pepper**

¼ **teaspoon red pepper flakes**

4 **cups chicken stock**

1 Place the beans in a large bowl and cover with 5 cups water. Allow to soak at room temperature 4–8 hours. Drain the beans and set aside.

2 Drizzle the oil into the Instant Pot®. Press the Sauté button and add the onion, carrots, and celery. Sauté until the vegetables are softened, about 5–6 minutes. Add the garlic and sauté an additional 30 seconds.

3 Add the salt, white pepper, red pepper flakes, and stock to the pot. Secure the lid.

4 Press the Manual or Pressure Cook button and adjust the time to 15 minutes.

5 When the timer beeps, let pressure release naturally until float valve drops and then unlock lid.

6 Allow to cool slightly before ladling into bowls to serve.

CALORIES: 372 | **FAT**: 10g | **PROTEIN**: 20g | **SODIUM**: 834mg
FIBER: 11g | **CARBOHYDRATES**: 51g | **SUGAR**: 8g

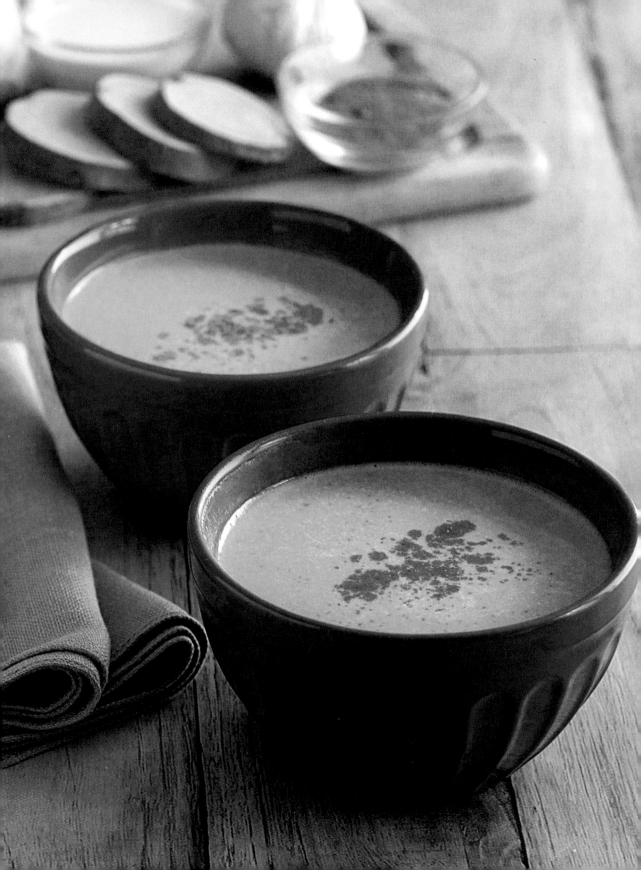

Coconut Curry Sweet Potato Soup

Coconut and curry are a match made in heaven in this creamy vegan soup. Full-fat canned coconut milk gives this delicious soup its rich and creamy texture without adding any dairy. Sweet potatoes are an excellent source of vitamins C and A and are known to help stabilize blood sugar levels, making them perfect for an anti-inflammatory diet.

- **Hands-On Time: 10 minutes**
- **Cook Time: 4 minutes**

Serves 4

1 tablespoon avocado oil

1 medium onion, peeled and diced

1 large sweet potato, peeled and cut into cubes

2 cloves garlic, minced

2 tablespoons mild curry powder

¼ teaspoon salt

¼ teaspoon black pepper

1 (13.25-ounce) can unsweetened full-fat coconut milk

4 cups vegetable broth

1 Press the Sauté button and heat the oil in the inner pot 1 minute. Add the onion and sauté 5 minutes.

2 Add the sweet potato, garlic, curry powder, salt, and pepper to the inner pot and sauté 1 minute more.

3 Add the coconut milk and broth and stir to combine. Secure the lid.

4 Press the Manual or Pressure Cook button and adjust the time to 4 minutes.

5 When the timer beeps, let pressure release naturally for 15 minutes, then quick-release any remaining pressure until float valve drops, then unlock lid.

6 Allow to cool slightly before ladling into bowls to serve.

CALORIES: 289 | **FAT:** 23g | **PROTEIN:** 3g | **SODIUM:** 712mg
FIBER: 4g | **CARBOHYDRATES:** 19g | **SUGAR:** 5g

Lentil Soup

Lentils are an amazing plant-based source of protein and iron, but many people have trouble digesting them. The great news is that you don't have to shy away from eating lentils. The Instant Pot® can help make lentils and other legumes more digestible! Pressure cooking increases the protein quality, destroys anti-nutrients like phytates and tannins, and deactivates lectins. This Lentil Soup is a nourishing vegan meal, full of vegetables and plant-based protein.

- **Hands-On Time: 15 minutes**
- **Cook Time: 24 minutes**

Serves 8

2 tablespoons avocado oil
½ medium yellow onion, peeled and diced
4 medium carrots, peeled and sliced
3 medium stalks celery, ends removed and sliced
1 tablespoon fresh thyme leaves
1 teaspoon paprika
1 teaspoon kosher salt
½ teaspoon black pepper
1½ cups dried brown lentils
2 teaspoons minced garlic
8 cups vegetable stock

1 Drizzle the oil into the Instant Pot®. Press the Sauté button and add the onion. Sauté the onion until it is softened and starting to brown, about 6 minutes.

2 Add the carrots, celery, thyme, paprika, salt, and pepper and continue to sauté until the vegetables are just softened, about 2 minutes.

3 Add the lentils and garlic to the Instant Pot® and stir to coat them in the spices. Cook another 30 seconds.

4 Add the stock and cover and seal the Instant Pot®.

5 Press the Cancel button and then the Manual or Pressure Cook button. Increase the time to 15 minutes.

6 When the timer beeps, let pressure release naturally for 10 minutes, then quick-release any remaining pressure until float valve drops, then unlock lid.

7 Serve warm.

CALORIES: 194 | **FAT**: 5g | **PROTEIN**: 12g | **SODIUM**: 1,190mg
FIBER: 5g | **CARBOHYDRATES**: 29g | **SUGAR**: 3g

Vegan Cauliflower Soup

The cruciferous vegetable family provides tremendous health benefits, and cauliflower is no exception. This vegan soup is made thick and creamy by blending half of it, while the unblended half provides bulk and a pleasing texture contrast. Fresh rosemary provides a lovely flavor, but if you don't have it, substitute 1 teaspoon dried rosemary.

- **Hands-On Time: 15 minutes**
- **Cook Time: 17 minutes**

Serves 6

1 tablespoon avocado oil

1 medium yellow onion, peeled and diced

1 clove garlic, minced

1 large head cauliflower, cored and chopped into large florets

2 sprigs fresh rosemary, tough stem removed and leaves chopped

1 teaspoon salt

¼ teaspoon black pepper

6 cups vegetable broth

1 Drizzle the oil into the Instant Pot®. Press the Sauté button and add the onion. Sauté the onion until it is softened and starting to brown, about 6 minutes.

2 Add the garlic and sauté an additional 30 seconds. Press the Cancel button.

3 Add the cauliflower, rosemary, salt, pepper, and broth and secure the lid. Press the Manual or Pressure Cook button and adjust the time to 10 minutes.

4 When the timer beeps, let pressure release naturally until float valve drops and then unlock lid.

5 Allow the soup to cool slightly, and then transfer half of the soup to a large blender and blend until smooth. Pour the blended soup back into the pot with the rest of the soup and stir to combine.

6 Allow to cool slightly before ladling into bowls to serve.

CALORIES: 78 | **FAT**: 3g | **PROTEIN**: 3g | **SODIUM**: 970mg
FIBER: 4g | **CARBOHYDRATES**: 12g | **SUGAR**: 4g

Butternut Squash and Apple Soup

Butternut squash has a natural sweetness that is offset by the tart apples in this recipe. Together with freshly grated nutmeg and bay leaf, you have flavors that scream "fall." You'll want to make this cozy soup weekly during the chilly autumn season, especially with only 8 minutes of cooking time!

- **Hands-On Time: 15 minutes**
- **Cook Time: 8 minutes**

Serves 8

1 large butternut squash, peeled, seeds removed, and cut into chunks

2 large green apples, peeled, cored, and cut into large chunks

1 teaspoon kosher salt

¼ teaspoon white pepper

¼ teaspoon freshly grated nutmeg

1 large bay leaf

8 cups vegetable stock

1 Place the squash, apples, salt, pepper, nutmeg, bay leaf, and stock in the inner pot of the Instant Pot®. Secure the lid.

2 Press the Manual or Pressure Cook button and adjust the time to 8 minutes.

3 When the timer beeps, let pressure release naturally until float valve drops and then unlock lid.

4 Allow the soup to cool slightly, and then transfer, in batches if necessary, to a large blender and blend until smooth. Alternatively, use an immersion blender to blend the soup to your desired consistency.

5 Allow to cool slightly before ladling into bowls to serve.

CALORIES: 74 | **FAT**: 1g | **PROTEIN**: 3g | **SODIUM**: 1,157mg
FIBER: 2g | **CARBOHYDRATES**: 17g | **SUGAR**: 8g

Turkey Chili

This unique chili recipe capitalizes on the smoky flavor of uncured turkey bacon along with smoked paprika and is hearty and filling with black beans and ground turkey. Don't skip the sliced avocado on top as it's the perfect contrasting texture and pairs perfectly with this mildly spicy bowl of chili.

- **Hands-On Time: 15 minutes**
- **Cook Time: 40 minutes**

Serves 8

- ½ **pound dry black beans**
- 10 **ounces uncured turkey bacon, chopped**
- ½ **large yellow onion, peeled and diced**
- 1 **pound lean ground turkey**
- 1 **tablespoon minced garlic**
- ½ **large red bell pepper, seeded and diced**
- ½ **large orange bell pepper, seeded and diced**
- 1 **medium jalapeño, seeded and minced**
- 2 **cups chicken stock**
- 1 **tablespoon dried oregano**
- 1 **teaspoon ground cumin**
- 2 **teaspoons kosher salt**
- 1 **teaspoon black pepper**
- 1 **teaspoon smoked paprika**
- 2 **tablespoons chili powder**
- 1 **tablespoon Worcestershire sauce**
- 1 **medium avocado, sliced**

1. Place the dry beans in a large bowl and cover with 5 cups water. Allow to soak at room temperature 4–8 hours. Drain the beans and set aside.

2. Press the Sauté button and use the Adjust tool to use the More setting. Add the bacon and sauté until crisp, stirring often, about 6–8 minutes. Transfer to a paper towel–lined plate.

3. Add the onion to the inner pot and sauté until just softened, about 3–4 minutes. Add the turkey and garlic and cook, stirring often until browned, about 7 minutes. Press the Cancel button.

4. Add the bell peppers, jalapeño, stock, oregano, cumin, salt, black pepper, paprika, chili powder, Worcestershire sauce, three-fourths of the cooked bacon, and the soaked beans. Scrape any brown bits from the bottom of the Instant Pot®. Secure the lid.

5. Press the Manual or Pressure Cook button and adjust the time to 25 minutes.

6. When the timer beeps, let pressure release naturally until float valve drops and then unlock lid. Serve each bowl with a little of the remaining bacon and avocado slices.

CALORIES: 295 | FAT: 6g | PROTEIN: 31g | SODIUM: 1,142mg
FIBER: 6g | CARBOHYDRATES: 25g | SUGAR: 3g

Beet Soup with Orange

Beets contain a class of antioxidants known as betalains, and that's what gives them strong anti-inflammatory properties. That's also where beets get their deep, vibrant hue that makes this soup a stunning addition to your table. The orange juice and orange zest added at the end are the perfect accompaniments to this soup as the sweetness balances beetroot's natural earthy flavor.

- **Hands-On Time: 10 minutes**
- **Cook Time: 15 minutes**

Serves 4

2 tablespoons avocado oil

5 small beets, peeled and chopped

1 medium yellow onion, peeled and chopped

1 teaspoon kosher salt

¼ teaspoon black pepper

4 cups vegetable broth

¼ cup fresh orange juice

1 tablespoon orange zest

1 Press the Sauté button, add the oil to the inner pot and allow it to heat 2 minutes.

2 Add the beets, onion, salt, and pepper and sauté 7 minutes. Press the Cancel button.

3 Add the broth and secure the lid. Press the Manual or Pressure Cook button and adjust the time to 8 minutes.

4 When the timer beeps, let pressure release naturally for 10 minutes, then quick-release any remaining pressure until float valve drops, then unlock lid.

5 Allow the soup to cool slightly, and then transfer, in batches if necessary, to a large blender and blend until smooth. Alternatively, use an immersion blender to blend the soup to your desired consistency. Stir in the orange juice and orange zest and serve.

CALORIES: 140 | FAT: 7g | PROTEIN: 2g | SODIUM: 1,202mg
FIBER: 5g | CARBOHYDRATES: 17g | SUGAR: 10g

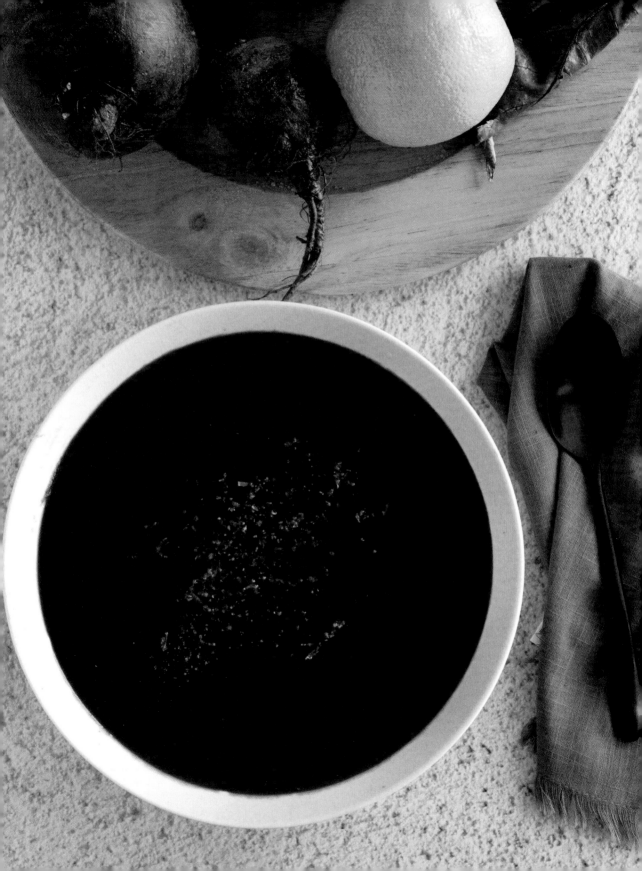

Creamy Mushroom Soup

You'll never believe that this creamy mushroom soup is actually made without any dairy at all. It's made with coconut milk, but you don't taste a hint of coconut in this savory soup. The mushrooms are the stars here, so if you're a mushroom lover, run, don't walk, to the kitchen to make this recipe.

- **Hands-On Time: 10 minutes**
- **Cook Time: 21 minutes**

Serves 4

2 tablespoons avocado oil

1 small yellow onion, peeled and chopped

8 ounces sliced white mushrooms

8 ounces sliced mini bella mushrooms

5 cloves garlic, minced

1 teaspoon kosher salt

½ teaspoon black pepper

1 (13.66-ounce) can unsweetened full-fat coconut milk

1 cup chicken stock

1 teaspoon dried oregano

1 Press the Sauté button and add the oil to the inner pot of the Instant Pot®. Allow it to heat 1 minute and then add the onion, mushrooms, garlic, salt, and pepper. Cook, stirring frequently until the mushrooms have cooked down and their liquid has released and evaporated, about 10 minutes. Press the Cancel button.

2 Add the coconut milk, stock, and oregano and stir to combine. Use a spoon to scrape any leftover brown bits from the bottom of the inner pot. Secure the lid.

3 Press the Manual or Pressure Cook button and adjust the time to 10 minutes.

4 When the timer beeps, let pressure release naturally until float valve drops and then unlock lid.

5 Allow to cool slightly before ladling into bowls to serve.

CALORIES: 155 | **FAT**: 13g | **PROTEIN**: 4g | **SODIUM**: 343mg
FIBER: 1g | **CARBOHYDRATES**: 6g | **SUGAR**: 2g

POWERFUL MUSHROOMS

Not only do mushrooms provide umami flavor that makes them irresistible, they are also packed with health benefits. Mushrooms are what's known as a prebiotic. This means they nourish the beneficial bacteria in your gut and help balance your microbiome.

"Cheesy" Broccoli Cauliflower Soup

No need to add dairy to your broccoli soup to get that satisfying cheesy flavor. Instead, we use a combination of vegetable stock and nutritional yeast. You'll be happily surprised at how well these two can work together to achieve a cheesy flavor and texture. All without the inflammatory effects dairy can have! The added cauliflower in this soup is a welcome bonus.

- **Hands-On Time: 20 minutes**
- **Cook Time: 8 minutes**

Serves 6

2 tablespoons avocado oil

1 medium yellow onion, peeled and chopped

3 medium carrots, peeled, ends removed and chopped

2 large stalks celery, ends removed and sliced

1 teaspoon kosher salt

½ teaspoon black pepper

1 medium head cauliflower, core removed and roughly chopped

3 small broccoli crowns, large stems removed and florets roughly chopped

8 cups vegetable stock

½ cup nutritional yeast

1 Press the Sauté button and add the oil to the inner pot of the Instant Pot®. Allow it to heat 1 minute and then add the onion, carrots, celery, salt, and pepper and sauté 5 minutes. Press the Cancel button.

2 Add the cauliflower, broccoli, stock, and nutritional yeast and stir to combine. Secure the lid.

3 Press the Manual or Pressure Cook button and adjust the time to 2 minutes.

4 When the timer beeps, let pressure release naturally until float valve drops and then unlock lid.

5 Allow to cool slightly before ladling into bowls to serve.

CALORIES: 154 | FAT: 6g | PROTEIN: 11g | SODIUM: 1,639mg
FIBER: 5g | CARBOHYDRATES: 19g | SUGAR: 5g

Three-Bean Chicken Chili

A flavorful chili with just 21 minutes cooking time sounds too good to be true, but it's not. This recipe saves time by used canned beans and even though it cooks quickly, the pressure cooking allows for a flavorful, full-bodied chili in a short amount of time. Three different beans means each one provides both a different nutritional profile as well as a different texture.

- **Hands-On Time: 10 minutes**
- **Cook Time: 21 minutes**

Serves 8

1 tablespoon avocado oil

1 large yellow onion, peeled and diced

2 medium carrots, peeled and diced

2 cloves garlic, minced

1 (15-ounce) can black beans, drained and rinsed

1 (15-ounce) can red kidney beans, drained and rinsed

1 (15-ounce) can pinto beans, drained and rinsed

1 tablespoon chili powder

1 teaspoon dried oregano

1 teaspoon salt

½ teaspoon black pepper

8 cups chicken stock

2 (5-ounce) boneless, skinless chicken breasts

1   Press the Sauté button and add the oil to the inner pot of the Instant Pot®. Allow it to heat 1 minute and then add the onion and carrots and sauté 5 minutes. Add the garlic and sauté another 5 minutes. Press the Cancel button.

2   Add the beans, chili powder, oregano, salt, pepper, and stock and stir to combine. Add the chicken breasts. Secure the lid.

3   Press the Manual or Pressure Cook button and adjust the time to 10 minutes.

4   When the timer beeps, let pressure release naturally until float valve drops and then unlock lid.

5   Use two forks to shred the chicken while it's still in the inner pot and then serve.

CALORIES: 295 | FAT: 5g | PROTEIN: 23g | SODIUM: 958mg
FIBER: 7g | CARBOHYDRATES: 36g | SUGAR: 6g

Golden Bone Broth

If two anti-inflammatory superpowers, bone broth and golden milk turmeric tea, had a baby, this is what you'd get. This recipe combines the nutritional benefits of bone broth with turmeric in one powerful punch. We start by making a turmeric paste and then add it to the bone broth mixture. This can be sipped on its own or used as a base for different soups that will complement a variety of flavors.

- **Hands-On Time: 10 minutes**
- **Cook Time: 90 minutes**

Serves 8

¼ cup turmeric powder
½ cup water
¾ teaspoon black pepper
½ teaspoon coconut oil
Bones from a 3–4 pound chicken
8 cups water
2 large carrots, cut into chunks
2 large stalks celery, ends removed and cut into chunks
1 large onion, peeled and cut into chunks
3 fresh rosemary sprigs
3 fresh thyme springs
2 tablespoons apple cider vinegar
1 teaspoon kosher salt

1 First, make your turmeric paste. Press the Sauté button and add the turmeric powder and water and stir until a paste is formed, then stir in the pepper. Press the Cancel button.

2 Add the rest of the ingredients to the inner pot and allow to sit 30 minutes.

3 Press the Manual or Pressure Cook button and adjust the time to 90 minutes.

4 When the timer beeps, let pressure release naturally until float valve drops and then unlock lid.

5 Strain the broth using a fine-mesh strainer and transfer into a storage container. Can be refrigerated three to five days or frozen up to six months.

CALORIES: 62 | FAT: 2g | PROTEIN: 8g | SODIUM: 313mg
FIBER: 1g | CARBOHYDRATES: 4g | SUGAR: 0g

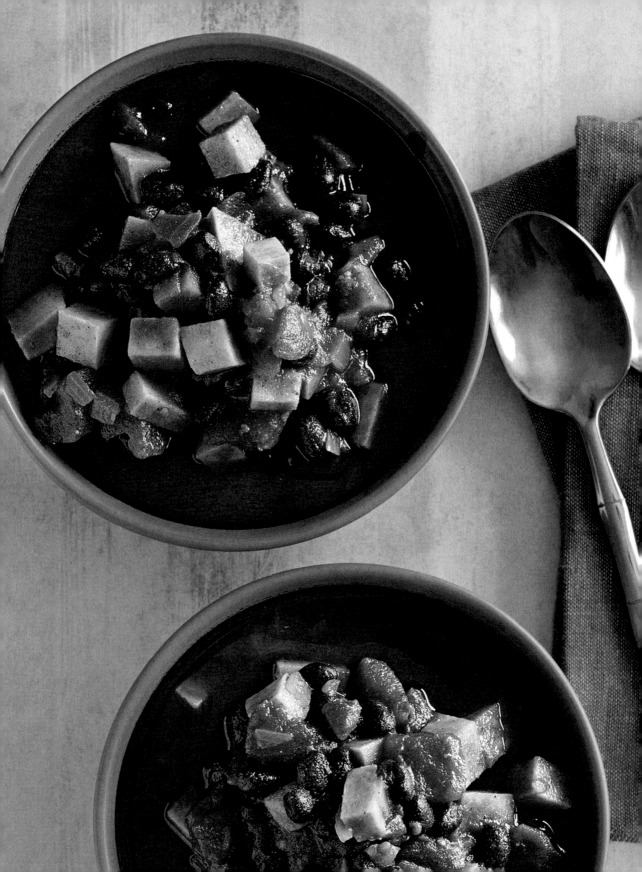

Sweet Potato Black Bean Chili

Southwest flavors are prevalent in this vegan chili. Ancho chili powder lends a subtle heat and smoked paprika adds a smoky depth that will leave you satisfied. Even meat lovers will be left wondering why they ever thought chili had to have beef to be amazing. The Instant Pot® makes this preparation so much quicker than the stovetop and pressure cooking intensifies the flavor.

- **Hands-On Time: 15 minutes**
- **Cook Time: 27 minutes**

Serves 6

½ pound dry black beans

1 tablespoon avocado oil

1 medium onion, peeled and diced

3 cloves garlic, minced

2 medium-large sweet potatoes, peeled and cut into 1" cubes

1½ tablespoons ancho chili powder

2 teaspoons ground cumin powder

1 teaspoon salt

¼ teaspoon black pepper

¼ teaspoon smoked paprika

¼ teaspoon ground cinnamon

1 (28-ounce) can diced fire-roasted tomatoes

3 cups vegetable stock

1 (6-ounce) can tomato paste

1 Place the dry beans in a large bowl and cover with 5 cups water. Allow to soak at room temperature 4–8 hours. Drain the beans and set aside.

2 Drizzle the oil into the Instant Pot®. Press the Sauté button, add the onion, and sauté until softened, about 5–6 minutes. Add the garlic and sauté an additional 30 seconds.

3 Add the soaked beans, sweet potatoes, chili powder, cumin, salt, pepper, paprika, cinnamon, tomatoes, stock, and tomato paste. Stir well to combine and scrape any brown bits from the bottom of the inner pot. Secure the lid.

4 Press the Manual or Pressure Cook button and adjust the time to 20 minutes.

5 When the timer beeps, let pressure release naturally for 10 minutes, then quick-release any remaining pressure until float valve drops, then unlock lid.

CALORIES: 268 | FAT: 4g | PROTEIN: 13g | SODIUM: 1,170mg
FIBER: 12g | CARBOHYDRATES: 49g | SUGAR: 17g

Vegetarian Unstuffed Cabbage Soup

This soup has all the flavors of traditional stuffed cabbage, but as a vegetarian soup. This is a hearty, filling soup that just happens to be packed with nutrition. Making stuffed cabbage rolls can be quite the process, but this soup could not be any easier and using the Instant Pot® is ideal for cooking the rice portion quickly.

- **Hands-On Time: 10 minutes**
- **Cook Time: 42 minutes**

Serves 6

1 tablespoon avocado oil

1 small yellow onion, peeled and chopped

8 ounces baby bella mushrooms

4 cloves garlic, minced

½ green cabbage, cored and cut into long slices (about 8 cups)

8 cups vegetable stock

1 (15-ounce) can diced tomatoes

1 cup short grain brown rice

1 teaspoon salt

1 teaspoon sweet paprika

1 Press the Sauté button, add the oil to the inner pot and allow it to heat 1 minute.

2 Add the onion and sauté 5 minutes. Add the mushrooms and continue to sauté until they are cooked down and their liquid has evaporated, about 7 minutes more.

3 Add the garlic and cook an additional 30 seconds.

4 Add the cabbage, stock, tomatoes, rice, salt, and paprika and stir to combine. Press the Cancel button.

5 Press the Manual or Pressure Cooker button and adjust the time to 28 minutes.

6 When the timer beeps, let pressure release naturally until float valve drops and then unlock lid.

7 Allow to cool slightly before ladling into bowls to serve.

CALORIES: 220 | FAT: 5g | PROTEIN: 8g | SODIUM: 1,697mg
FIBER: 5g | CARBOHYDRATES: 40g | SUGAR: 8g

Vegan Split Pea Soup

Split peas are an excellent source of plant-based protein and also provide a good amount of fiber, copper, folate, and vitamin B_1 to your diet. There's no need to add ham to your split pea soup to get that classic smoky flavor, smoked paprika gets the job done brilliantly!

- **Hands-On Time: 10 minutes**
- **Cook Time: 23 minutes**

Serves 8

¼ cup avocado oil

1 large leek, white and light green parts, cut in half, washed well, and thinly sliced into half moons

1 medium onion, peeled and finely chopped

3 medium carrots, peeled and sliced

3 medium stalks celery, ends removed and thinly sliced

3 cloves garlic, minced

1 teaspoon fine sea salt

½ teaspoon black pepper

1 pound dried green split peas, picked over and rinsed

1 teaspoon dried thyme

1 teaspoon smoked paprika

8 cups vegetable broth

2 tablespoons fresh lemon juice

1 Press the Sauté button and add the oil to the inner pot. Allow it to heat 1 minute and then add the leek, onion, carrots, celery, and garlic and cook, stirring frequently until the vegetables are softened, about 8–10 minutes. Press the Cancel button.

2 Add the rest of the ingredients, except the lemon juice, and stir to combine. Secure the lid.

3 Press the Manual or Pressure Cook button and adjust the time to 12 minutes.

4 When the timer beeps, let pressure release naturally until float valve drops and then unlock lid. Stir in the lemon juice.

5 Use an immersion blender to blend until the desired consistency is achieved and then serve.

CALORIES: 373 | **FAT**: 10g | **PROTEIN**: 20g | **SODIUM**: 577mg
FIBER: 16g | **CARBOHYDRATES**: 51g | **SUGAR**: 11g

Turkey and Wild Rice Stew

Thick and hearty, this is one of the most flavorful and satisfying stews you will ever make. Filled with nourishing vegetables, herbs, a nutty wild rice blend, and lean ground turkey, this one will have you forgetting that you're eating healthy food. Don't skip the sliced almonds, as they provide an interesting contrasting texture that makes this stew extra special.

- **Hands-On Time: 10 minutes**
- **Cook Time: 36 minutes**

Serves 6

1 tablespoon avocado oil

1 medium yellow onion, peeled and diced

2 medium carrots, peeled and chopped

2 medium stalks celery, ends removed and sliced

8 ounces sliced white mushrooms

4 cloves garlic, minced

1 tablespoon Worcestershire sauce

1 teaspoon dried thyme

1 teaspoon dried rosemary

1 teaspoon salt

¼ teaspoon black pepper

1 pound lean ground turkey

4 cups chicken stock

1 cup wild rice blend

½ cup sliced almonds

1. Press the Sauté button and add the oil to the inner pot and let it heat 1 minute. Add the onion, carrots, celery, mushrooms, garlic, Worcestershire sauce, thyme, rosemary, salt, and pepper and sauté 10 minutes. Add the turkey and sauté an additional 5 minutes. Press the Cancel button.

2. Add the stock and rice and stir. Secure the lid.

3. Press the Manual or Pressure Cook button and adjust the time to 20 minutes.

4. When the timer beeps, let pressure release naturally for 10 minutes, then quick-release any remaining pressure until float valve drops, then unlock lid.

5. Stir in the sliced almonds and serve.

CALORIES: 362 | **FAT:** 14g | **PROTEIN:** 26g | **SODIUM:** 725mg
FIBER: 4g | **CARBOHYDRATES:** 34g | **SUGAR:** 7g

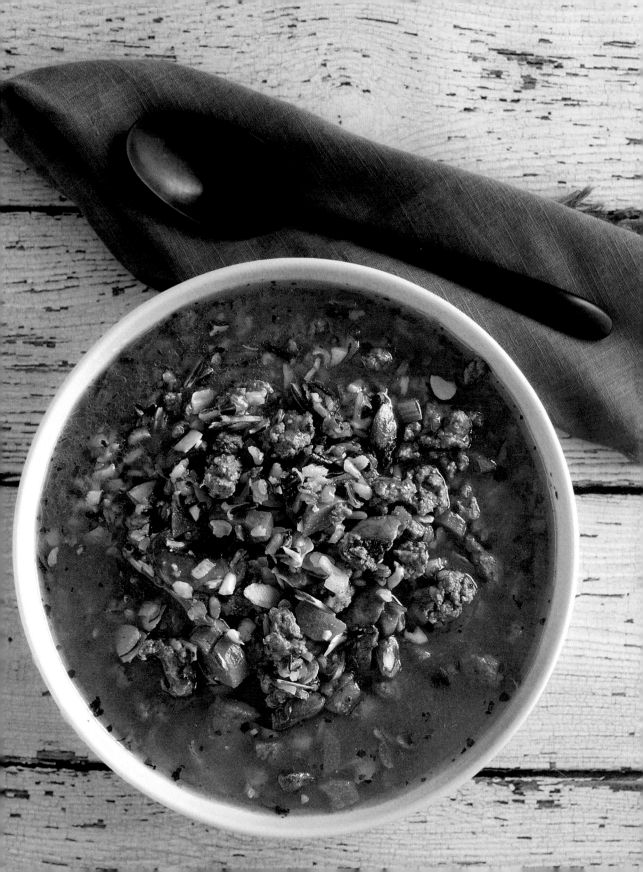

Snacks and Appetizers

Whenever you're super hungry in between meals, do you reach for pre-packaged food? Sometimes it just seems quicker and easier than opting for something fresh. You aren't alone. The snack aisle at the supermarket is one of the most-traveled aisles in the store, and unfortunately you can't always find the most nutritious options there.

Snacks and appetizers can pose the biggest challenge when eating an anti-inflammatory diet. So many of the popular snacks and appetizers of mainstream diets are made with inflammatory ingredients. So many snacks are made with added sugars, refined flours, and hydrogenated oils. The appetizer menu is often filled with options that are either deep fried or loaded with dairy, and finding anything with a vegetable is difficult.

In this chapter, you'll find a myriad of recipes filled with nutrient-dense, inflammatory-fighting foods that will satisfy your hunger and your taste buds. As an added bonus, the Instant Pot® takes a lot of the fuss out of cooking these homemade snacks and appetizers.

From kid-friendly homemade applesauce and granola bars to party-ready appetizers like Sweet Potato Hummus and Vegan Spinach Artichoke Dip, you'll find exactly what you need in this chapter!

Cinnamon Applesauce

Making homemade applesauce could not be easier than it is in the Instant Pot®. There's no need to peel the apples as a powerful blender will yield a smooth sauce and the peels add nutrients. For a sweeter applesauce, use sweeter apples like Fuji, Golden Delicious, or Gala. For less sweet, use a mix of apples and add a tart variety such as Macintosh or Granny Smith.

- **Hands-On Time: 10 minutes**
- **Cook Time: 5 minutes**

Serves 12

4 pounds apples, cored and cut into pieces
¼ cup water
2 teaspoons lemon juice
2 teaspoons ground cinnamon

1 Place the apples, water, lemon juice, and cinnamon in the Instant Pot®. Stir to combine. Secure the lid.

2 Press the Manual or Pressure Cook button and set time to 5 minutes.

3 When the timer beeps, let pressure release naturally for 10 minutes, then quick-release any remaining pressure until float valve drops, then unlock lid.

4 Transfer the apples (including the liquid) to a large blender and blend on high until desired consistency is achieved.

5 Allow to cool and then store in airtight containers. Will keep refrigerated seven to ten days. May be frozen up to two months.

CALORIES: 67 | **FAT**: 0g | **PROTEIN**: 0g | **SODIUM**: 1mg
FIBER: 3g | **CARBOHYDRATES**: 18g | **SUGAR**: 13g

Chewy Cinnamon Raisin Granola Bars

Store-bought granola bars can be filled with unwanted ingredients, including refined sugar, high-fructose corn syrup, and hydrogenated oils. You can avoid all of these by making your own homemade granola bars at home. The Instant Pot® keeps it super simple; it's as easy as mixing your ingredients in one bowl and cooking inside the pot. This recipe yields a soft, chewy granola bar with warm cinnamon flavors spiked with soft raisins. These are the perfect, satisfying snack.

- **Hands-On Time: 10 minutes**
- **Cook Time: 10 minutes**

Serves 10

2 cups quick-cooking oats
⅓ cup date syrup
⅓ cup avocado oil
⅓ cup monk fruit sweetener
⅓ cup almond butter
⅓ cup raisins
½ teaspoon ground cinnamon

1 In a medium bowl, combine the oats, date syrup, oil, sweetener, almond butter, raisins, and cinnamon.

2 Spray a 5" baking dish with cooking spray. Press the oat mixture firmly into the pan.

3 Add 1 cup water to the inner pot and place the steam rack inside. Place the baking dish on top of the steam rack. Secure the lid.

4 Press the Manual or Pressure Cook button and adjust the time to 10 minutes.

5 When the timer beeps, quick-release pressure until float valve drops and then unlock lid.

6 Carefully remove the pan from the inner pot and place it on a baking rack to cool completely. Once completely cooled, turn the pan upside down onto a cutting board to remove the granola from the pan. Cut into ten bars.

CALORIES: 222 | **FAT**: 12g | **PROTEIN**: 4g | **SODIUM**: 7mg
FIBER: 3g | **CARBOHYDRATES**: 30g | **SUGAR**: 11g

Chewy Almond Butter Chocolate Chip Granola Bars

Sometimes, it's a happy accident when your healthy snack tastes like a candy bar. Nobody will complain that the anti-inflammatory diet is restrictive or lacking in any way once they've tried these bars. Almond butter and stevia-sweetened chocolate chips make these chewy granola bars taste way more indulgent than they actually are.

- **Hands-On Time: 10 minutes**
- **Cook Time: 10 minutes**

Serves 10

2 cups quick-cooking oats
⅔ cup almond butter
⅓ cup avocado oil
⅓ cup monk fruit sweetener
⅓ cup stevia-sweetened dark chocolate chips
¼ teaspoon salt

ALMOND BUTTER SUBSTITUTION IDEAS
While almond butter is delicious, it won't work for anyone allergic to tree nuts. If that's you or a family member, consider using an unsweetened sunflower seed butter for this recipe and the substitution is one to one.

1. In a medium bowl, combine the oats, almond butter, oil, sweetener, chocolate chips, and salt.

2. Spray a 5" baking dish with cooking spray. Press the oat mixture firmly into the pan.

3. Add 1 cup water to the inner pot and place the steam rack inside. Place the baking dish on top of the steam rack. Secure the lid.

4. Press the Manual or Pressure Cook button and adjust the time to 10 minutes.

5. When the timer beeps, quick-release pressure until float valve drops and then unlock lid.

6. Carefully remove the pan from the inner pot and place it on a baking rack to cool completely. Once completely cooled, turn the pan upside down onto a cutting board to remove the granola from the pan. Cut into ten bars.

CALORIES: 254 | **FAT**: 19g | **PROTEIN**: 6g | **SODIUM**: 60mg
FIBER: 5g | **CARBOHYDRATES**: 25g | **SUGAR**: 3g

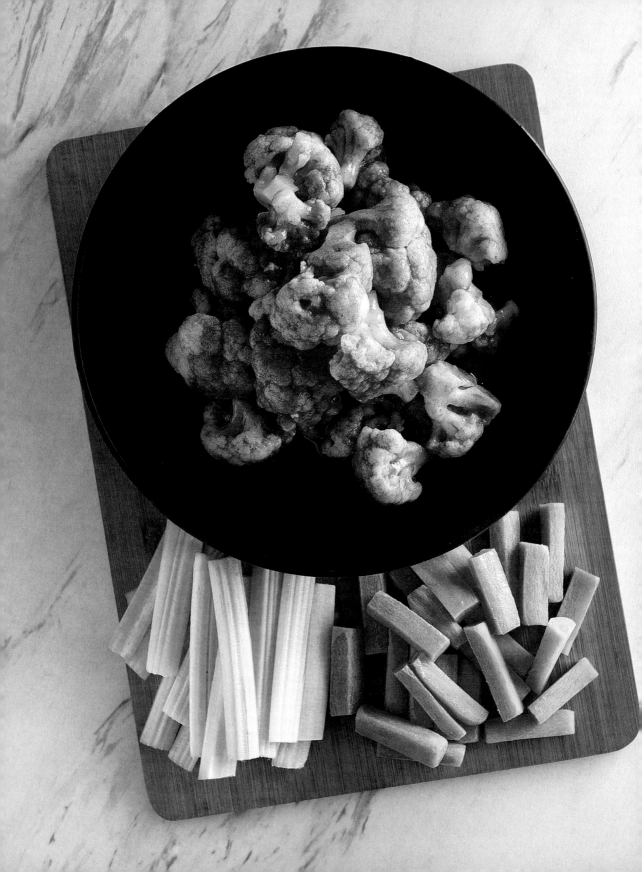

Buffalo Cauliflower Bites (pictured)

You'll forget about chicken wings when you try these spicy buffalo-flavored cauliflower bites. They have all the flavor, but with the added bonus of all the nutritional benefits of cauliflower.

- **Hands-On Time: 5 minutes**
- **Cook Time: 2 minutes**

Serves 4

1 large head cauliflower, cut into large pieces
½ cup buffalo hot sauce

1 Pour 1 cup water into the Instant Pot® and place the steam rack inside.

2 Place the cauliflower in a 7-cup glass bowl and add the buffalo hot sauce. Toss to evenly coat. Place the bowl on top of the steam rack. Secure the lid.

3 Press the Manual or Pressure Cook button and adjust the time to 2 minutes.

4 When the timer beeps, quick-release pressure until float valve drops and then unlock lid.

5 Transfer to a plate and serve with toothpicks.

CALORIES: 52 | FAT: 0g | PROTEIN: 4g | SODIUM: 982mg
FIBER: 4g | CARBOHYDRATES: 10g | SUGAR: 4g

Vegan Nacho Cheese Sauce

Right when you thought your days of enjoying nacho cheese sauce were over, you found this vegan recipe. Serve this sauce with grain-free tortilla chips or oven-baked vegetable chips.

- **Hands-On Time: 5 minutes**
- **Cook Time: 10 minutes**

Serves 4

1¼ cups vegetable broth
1 cup plain nondairy yogurt
3 tablespoons oat flour
¼ teaspoon salt
¼ teaspoon garlic salt
½ teaspoon cumin
1 teaspoon chili powder
¼ teaspoon paprika
⅛ teaspoon cayenne powder

1 Press the Sauté button and use the Adjust button to set the More setting. Add the broth to the inner pot and let it come to a boil.

2 Meanwhile, in a small bowl, mix together the yogurt and flour. Stir until well combined.

3 Use the Adjust button to change the Sauté setting to Normal.

4 Add the yogurt mixture, salt, and spices to the pot and cook and stir until thick and bubbly, about 5 minutes. Transfer to a bowl and serve.

CALORIES: 64 | FAT: 1g | PROTEIN: 2g | SODIUM: 464mg
FIBER: 1g | CARBOHYDRATES: 10g | SUGAR: 3g

Dairy-Free Buffalo Chicken Dip

This recipe proves that eating an anti-inflammatory diet doesn't have to mean deprivation. It is as much about eliminating inflammatory foods like dairy as it is about eating foods that help fight inflammation. This Dairy-Free Buffalo Chicken Dip is a great way to enjoy a favorite party food while still sticking to your anti-inflammatory regimen. You will be shocked that there's no dairy in this recipe!

- **Hands-On Time: 5 minutes**
- **Cook Time: 7 minutes**

Serves 10

2 cups cooked, shredded chicken
1 cup vegan nondairy blue cheese-style dressing
8 ounces nondairy cream cheese
½ cup buffalo hot sauce

BE A SMART SHOPPER

Not all nondairy products you can buy in the supermarket are created equally. Look for ones that are made with clean ingredients and no inflammatory oils. Sometimes you have to search, but they are out there!

1 In a 7" glass bowl, add the chicken, blue cheese dressing, cream cheese, and hot sauce. Mix until well combined.

2 Add 1 cup water to the inner pot and place the steam rack inside. Place the bowl on top of the steam rack. Secure the lid.

3 Press the Manual or Pressure Cook button and adjust the time to 7 minutes.

4 When the timer beeps, let pressure release naturally until float valve drops and then unlock lid.

5 Stir the dip and then serve warm.

CALORIES: 210 | **FAT**: 17g | **PROTEIN**: 8g | **SODIUM**: 738mg
FIBER: 0g | **CARBOHYDRATES**: 5g | **SUGAR**: 1g

Vegan Spinach Artichoke Dip

This appetizer is so simple to create: just put the ingredients into the Instant Pot®. Serve this with grain-free tortilla chips or vegetable crudités.

- **Hands-On Time: 5 minutes**
- **Cook Time: 6 minutes**

Serves 10

½ cup vegetable stock

1 (10-ounce) package frozen, cut spinach (does not need to be thawed)

1 (14-ounce) can artichoke quarters, drained

8 ounces nondairy cream cheese

¾ cup nondairy Greek yogurt

¼ cup vegan mayonnaise

1 teaspoon onion powder

¼ teaspoon garlic salt

¼ teaspoon black pepper

1 cup nutritional yeast

1 Add all of the ingredients to the inner pot of the Instant Pot®. Secure the lid.

2 Press the Manual or Pressure Cook button and adjust the time to 6 minutes.

3 When the timer beeps, quick-release pressure until float valve drops and then unlock lid.

4 Stir well and then transfer the dip to a serving bowl. The dip will thicken as it sits.

CALORIES: 163 | FAT: 11g | PROTEIN: 7g | SODIUM: 402mg
FIBER: 4g | CARBOHYDRATES: 11g | SUGAR: 6g

Sweet Potato Hummus

Traditional hummus gets an extra nutritional boost from vitamin A–rich sweet potatoes in this healthy appetizer. The sweetness of the potatoes is countered nicely with the sesame paste and ground cumin. A perfect balance! To keep this an anti-inflammatory snack, use this hummus as a dip for carrot sticks, celery stalks, or cucumbers.

- **Hands-On Time: 10 minutes**
- **Cook Time: 7 minutes**

Serves 10

2 tablespoons avocado oil

1 large sweet potato, peeled and cut into cubes

½ teaspoon salt

3 cloves garlic, minced

Juice from 1 large lemon

1 (15-ounce) can cooked chickpeas

¼ cup tahini

1 teaspoon ground cumin

A SWEET VERSION
While this savory recipe is delicious as is, it is also tasty when taken in a sweet direction. Eliminate the garlic and use cinnamon in the place of cumin, then add a touch of maple syrup.

1 Press the Sauté button and pour the oil into the inner pot. Allow it to heat 2 minutes.

2 Add the sweet potato and salt and sauté 2 minutes. Add the garlic and sauté an additional 30 seconds. Press the Cancel button.

3 Add the lemon juice and secure the lid. Press the Manual or Pressure Cook button and adjust the time to 2 minutes.

4 When the timer beeps, quick-release pressure until float valve drops and then unlock lid. Allow the mixture to cool.

5 Transfer the contents of the inner pot to a large food processor. Add the chickpeas, tahini, and cumin and process until you have a smooth mixture.

6 Allow the hummus to chill in the refrigerator at least 30 minutes before serving.

CALORIES: 114 | **FAT**: 6g | **PROTEIN**: 4g | **SODIUM**: 250mg
FIBER: 3g | **CARBOHYDRATES**: 11g | **SUGAR**: 1g

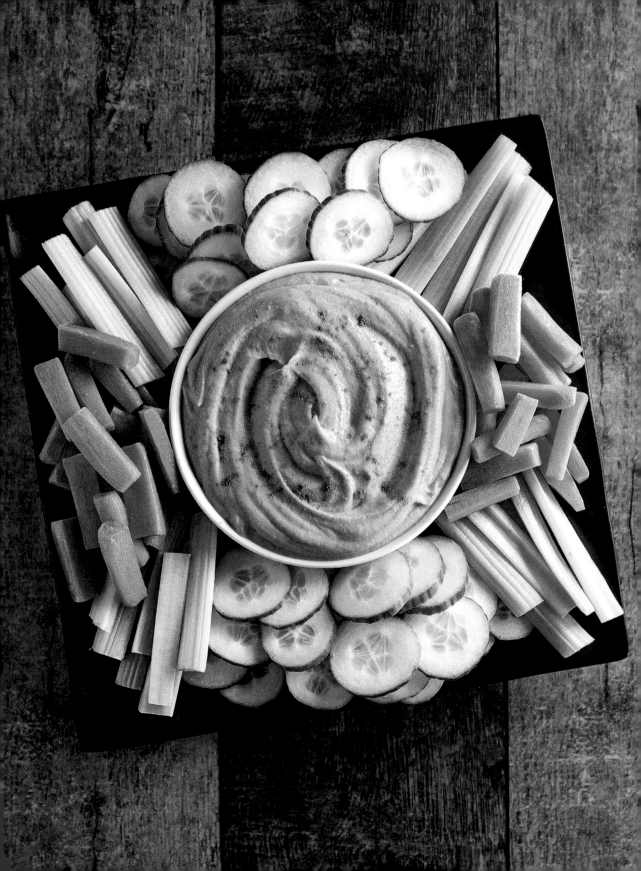

Cauliflower Hummus

There isn't much cauliflower can't do, and that list includes being cooked and whipped into a party-worthy hummus. If you've already tried cauliflower pizza crust, cauliflower rice, and cauliflower "chicken wings," it's time to give cauliflower hummus a turn. Cauliflower whips up beautifully smooth in this creamy hummus recipe.

- **Hands-On Time: 15 minutes**
- **Cook Time: 14 minutes**

Serves 10

1 tablespoon avocado oil

1 small yellow onion, chopped

3 cloves garlic, minced

1 small head cauliflower, cut into florets

¾ cup water

½ teaspoon salt

Juice from 1 large lemon

1 (15-ounce) can cooked chickpeas

¼ cup tahini

1 teaspoon ground cumin

1 Press the Sauté button and pour the oil into the inner pot. Allow it to heat 1 minute.

2 Add the onion and sauté 7 minutes until the onion is soft and starting to brown. Add the garlic and sauté an additional 30 seconds. Press the Cancel button.

3 Add the cauliflower and water and secure the lid. Press the Manual or Pressure Cook button and adjust the time to 5 minutes.

4 When the timer beeps, quick-release pressure until float valve drops and then unlock lid. Allow the mixture to cool.

5 Transfer the contents of the inner pot to a large food processor, except the liquid. Add the salt, lemon juice, chickpeas, tahini, and cumin and process until you have a smooth mixture. If the mixture is too thick, add some of the liquid from the inner pot until it is the consistency you prefer.

6 Allow the hummus to chill in the refrigerator at least 30 minutes before serving.

CALORIES: 97 | FAT: 5g | PROTEIN: 4g | SODIUM: 253mg
FIBER: 3g | CARBOHYDRATES: 10g | SUGAR: 1g

Smoky Black Bean Dip

Black beans are a great source of nutrients like zinc, folate, copper, magnesium, and iron. They just happen to blend up beautifully to create this smoky, complex dip that is as flavorful as it is nutritious. This dip is delicious served warm, but it can also be eaten at room temperature.

- **Hands-On Time: 5 minutes**
- **Cook Time: 7 minutes**

Serves 10

1 tablespoon avocado oil

1 medium yellow onion, peeled and chopped

2 (15-ounce) cans black beans, drained and rinsed

1 teaspoon ground cumin

½ teaspoon chili powder

½ teaspoon smoked paprika

½ teaspoon salt

Juice from ½ medium lime

¼ cup nutritional yeast

MAKE IT A MEAL

Even though this is a recipe for an appetizer, this tasty dip can be made into a meal. Spread it on a large romaine lettuce leaf and top with grilled onions, tomatoes, and avocado for a terrific lunch.

1 Press the Sauté button and add the oil to the inner pot. Let it heat 1 minute and then add the onion. Sauté the onion, stirring occasionally until softened, about 3 minutes. Press the Cancel button.

2 Add the beans, cumin, chili powder, paprika, and salt. Secure the lid.

3 Press the Manual or Pressure Cook button and adjust the timer to 3 minutes.

4 When the timer beeps, quick-release pressure until float valve drops and then unlock lid.

5 Add the lime juice and nutritional yeast and use an immersion blender to blend the dip to a chunky consistency. Serve warm.

CALORIES: 100 | FAT: 2g | PROTEIN: 6g | SODIUM: 313mg
FIBER: 6g | CARBOHYDRATES: 16g | SUGAR: 1g

White Bean Basil Dip

Fresh basil brings its outstanding, bright flavor to this easy appetizer. Cannelloni beans make a nutritious base for this dip, and they also provide a natural creaminess. While this mixture makes a lovely dip, you can also use this as a sandwich spread for your favorite vegetable sandwich.

- **Hands-On Time: 5 minutes**
- **Cook Time: 8 minutes**

Serves 10

1 tablespoon avocado oil

1 medium yellow onion, peeled and chopped

2 cloves garlic, minced

2 (15-ounce) cans cannelloni beans, drained and rinsed

1 (15-ounce) can diced tomatoes, drained

½ teaspoon salt

¼ teaspoon black pepper

½ cup chopped fresh basil

1 tablespoon fresh lemon juice

1 Press the Sauté button and add the oil to the inner pot. Let it heat 1 minute and then add the onion. Sauté the onion, stirring occasionally until softened, about 3 minutes. Add the garlic and sauté an additional 30 seconds. Press the Cancel button.

2 Add the beans, tomatoes, salt, and pepper and stir to combine. Secure the lid.

3 Press the Manual or Pressure Cook button and adjust the time to 3 minutes.

4 When the timer beeps, quick-release pressure until float valve drops and then unlock lid.

5 Stir in the basil and lemon juice and then use an immersion blender to blend to a chunky consistency. Serve warm or cold.

CALORIES: 84 | **FAT**: 1g | **PROTEIN**: 5g | **SODIUM**: 362mg
FIBER: 6g | **CARBOHYDRATES**: 16g | **SUGAR**: 2g

Edamame

Edamame are whole, immature soybeans and are sold both encased in their pods or already shelled. The steamer function cooks the beans from frozen to ready to eat in just 1 minute.

- **Hands-On Time: 1 minute**
- **Cook Time: 1 minute**

Serves 4

1 (10-ounce) bag frozen edamame in pods
2 tablespoons reduced sodium tamari
¼ teaspoon kosher salt

1 Place 1 cup water in the inner pot and place a steam rack in the pot.

2 Place the edamame in a steamer basket and place basket on top of the steam rack.

3 Press the Steam button and adjust the time to 1 minute.

4 When the timer beeps, quick-release pressure until float valve drops and then unlock lid.

5 Transfer the edamame to a medium bowl and top with the tamari and salt and serve.

CALORIES: 84 | FAT: 0g | PROTEIN: 8g | SODIUM: 366mg
FIBER: 3g | CARBOHYDRATES: 7g | SUGAR: 2g

Warm Cinnamon Almonds

Almonds are nutritious nuts that make a great snack. These are irresistible served warm, but they can also be eaten at room temperature.

- **Hands-On Time: 2 minutes**
- **Cook Time: 2 minutes**

Serves 8

2 cups raw unsalted almonds
1 teaspoon ground cinnamon
2 tablespoons water
40 drops pure liquid stevia
½ teaspoon pure vanilla extract
¼ teaspoon coarse salt

1 Place all the ingredients into a 7-cup glass bowl and toss to combine.

2 Pour ½ cup hot water into the Instant Pot® and place the steam rack inside. Place the bowl with the almonds on top of the rack. Secure the lid.

3 Press the Manual or Pressure Cook button and adjust the time to 2 minutes.

4 When the timer beeps, quick-release pressure until float valve drops and then unlock lid. Serve warm.

CALORIES: 161 | FAT: 14g | PROTEIN: 6g | SODIUM: 48mg
FIBER: 3g | CARBOHYDRATES: 6g | SUGAR: 1g

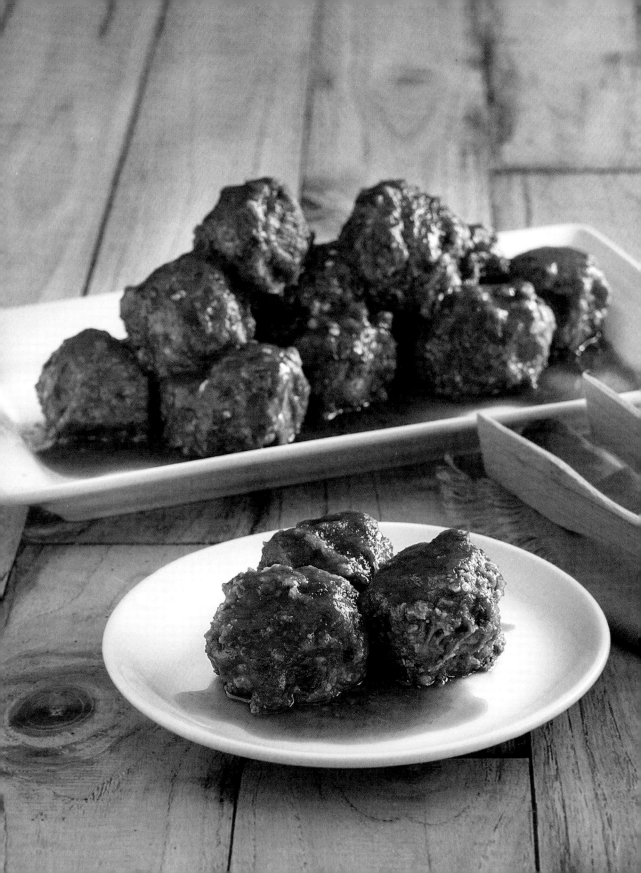

Comforting Lentil Balls

With black beans and lentils, there is plenty of protein in this meatless appetizer, and the flavor is deep and addicting. They're sure to be a party hit!

- **Hands-On Time: 40 minutes**
- **Cook Time: 13 minutes**

Serves 4/Yields 12–15 balls

For the Lentil Balls
⅓ cup cooked black beans, drained and rinsed
½ cup old fashioned rolled oats
1¼ cups cooked lentils
¼ cup unsweetened almond milk
¼ teaspoon coarse salt
¼ teaspoon ground ginger
⅛ teaspoon garlic powder
⅛ teaspoon black pepper
2 tablespoons avocado oil
2 tablespoons oat flour

For the Sauce
¾ cup tomato sauce
1 tablespoon tomato paste
¼ cup maple syrup
2 tablespoons cup coconut aminos
1 tablespoon apple cider vinegar
½ teaspoon ground ginger
¼ teaspoon crushed red pepper flakes

1. **To make Lentil Balls:** In a medium bowl partially mash the black beans.

2. In a food processor pulse the oats a few times. Add the lentils and pulse again. Add the milk, salt, ginger, garlic powder, and pepper and pulse. Do not over mix.

3. Combine the lentil mixture and black beans, stirring well. Form into tablespoon-sized balls and refrigerate 30 minutes.

4. **To make the Sauce:** Mix all of the sauce ingredients together in a medium bowl.

5. Press the Sauté button, then Adjust button to change setting to More. Add the avocado oil to the inner pot. Allow it to heat 2 minutes.

6. Place the oat flour in a shallow bowl and dredge each lentil ball in the flour to coat it.

7. Add the lentil balls to the oil and carefully move them around to brown, about 1 minute per side. Press the Cancel button.

8. Remove the balls and place them inside a 6" cake pan. Cover with the sauce and a paper towel, then cover tightly with foil.

9. Add ½ cup water to inner pot and scrape up any brown bits from the bottom. Place the steam rack in the pot and the pan of lentil balls on top of it. Secure the lid.

10. Press the Manual or Pressure Cook button and adjust the time to 5 minutes.

11. When the timer beeps, quick-release pressure until float valve drops and unlock lid. Carefully remove the pan and serve.

CALORIES: 288 | FAT: 8g | PROTEIN: 10g | SODIUM: 576mg
FIBER: 9g | CARBOHYDRATES: 44g | SUGAR: 16g

Quinoa Almond Butter Energy Balls

Quinoa has a mostly neutral flavor, but provides a great base of protein and nutrients for these unique energy balls. Almond butter and honey lend an irresistible flavor that kids and adults both enjoy. The blackstrap molasses adds a depth of flavor and also plant-based iron to these nutritious snack balls.

- **Hands-On Time: 15 minutes**
- **Cook Time: 1 minute**

Yields 20 balls

½ cup quinoa
1 cup water
¼ cup almond butter
2 teaspoons raw honey
½ teaspoon ground cinnamon
½ teaspoon blackstrap molasses
⅛ teaspoon fine sea salt

GETTING ENOUGH PROTEIN?

Quinoa is one of only a few plant-based sources that provide a complete protein. It's a great way to add protein to your diet if you have trouble getting enough on a daily basis.

1 Place the quinoa in a fine-mesh strainer and rinse under water until the water runs clear.

2 Add the quinoa and water to the inner pot. Secure the lid.

3 Press the Manual or Pressure Cook button and adjust the time to 1 minute.

4 When the timer beeps, quick-release pressure until float valve drops and then unlock lid.

5 Transfer the cooked quinoa to a medium bowl and allow it to cool. Once it is cooled, add the rest of the ingredients to the bowl and stir to combine.

6 Form the mixture into 1" balls and place them onto a tray or plate. Place them in the freezer about 30 minutes to firm. Keep stored in the refrigerator.

CALORIES: 37 | **FAT**: 2g | **PROTEIN**: 1g | **SODIUM**: 10mg
FIBER: 1g | **CARBOHYDRATES**: 4g | **SUGAR**: 1g

Broccoli Sesame Bites

Why have a vegetable tray at your party when you can make your vegetables more interesting? Broccoli is treated with Asian flavors in this simple hot appetizer. With minimal prep time and 1 minute cooking time, it's worth adding this to your party food menu. Of course the fact that broccoli is loaded with anti-inflammatory properties is just an added bonus.

- **Hands-On Time: 7 minutes**
- **Cook Time: 1 minute**

Serves 4

1 large crown broccoli, cut into large pieces
2 tablespoons toasted sesame oil
½ teaspoon salt
¼ teaspoon ground ginger
⅛ teaspoon garlic powder
2 tablespoons sesame seeds

1 Place the broccoli pieces into a 6" cake pan.

2 In a small bowl, whisk together the oil, salt, ginger, and garlic powder. Add it to the broccoli and toss to coat.

3 Pour 1 cup water into the Instant Pot® and place the steam rack inside. Place the pan with broccoli on top of the steam rack. Secure the lid.

4 Press the Manual or Pressure Cook button and adjust the time to 1 minute.

5 When the timer beeps, quick-release pressure until float valve drops and then unlock lid. Carefully remove the pan from the inner pot.

6 Add the sesame seeds to the broccoli and toss to coat. Transfer to a plate and serve with toothpicks.

CALORIES: 103 | **FAT**: 9g | **PROTEIN**: 3g | **SODIUM**: 307mg
FIBER: 1g | **CARBOHYDRATES**: 4g | **SUGAR**: 0g

Perfect Hard-Boiled Eggs

Hard-boiled eggs are not difficult to make on the stovetop, but they are difficult to have turn out perfectly every time. Furthermore, peeling hard-boiled eggs made on the stovetop is no easy task. The Instant Pot® is a game-changer when it comes to hard-boiled eggs. They come out perfectly every time with no guesswork, and the shells peel away easily. You'll never boil eggs on the stove again!

- **Hands-On Time: 2 minutes**
- **Cook Time: 7 minutes**

Serves 6

6 large eggs

1 Pour 1 cup water into the inner pot of your Instant Pot® and place the steam rack inside.

2 Carefully place the eggs directly onto the steam rack.

3 Press the Steam button and adjust the time to 7 minutes.

4 When the timer beeps, quick-release pressure until float valve drops and then unlock lid.

5 Immediately transfer the eggs to a bowl filled with iced water and let them sit 15 minutes.

6 Remove the eggs from the water and peel the shells away from the eggs. Store in the refrigerator.

CALORIES: 77 | **FAT**: 4g | **PROTEIN**: 6g | **SODIUM**: 62mg
FIBER: 0g | **CARBOHYDRATES**: 1g | **SUGAR**: 1g

Simple Avocado Hummus

If you aren't crazy about tahini or just never keep it in the house, give this Simple Avocado Hummus a try. It's made without any tahini, and is super creamy thanks to the fat content in the nutritional powerhouse avocado. Olive oil and lemon juice are also added, which lend complementary flavors. Top your hummus with a sprinkle of crushed red pepper for just a little kick.

- **Hands-On Time: 10 minutes**
- **Cook Time: 10 minutes**

Serves 8

¾ cup dry chickpeas

3 cups water

1 teaspoon salt

1 large avocado, peeled, pitted, and sliced

2 tablespoons extra-virgin olive oil plus ⅛ teaspoon for drizzling

2 tablespoons fresh lemon juice

½ teaspoon crushed red pepper flakes

A SNACK AND A CONDIMENT
Hummus makes a favorite dipping snack, but it is also wonderful as a condiment. Use it as a spread for wraps and sandwiches or thin it with water and use it as a salad dressing!

1 Put the chickpeas in a bowl and cover with 3" water. Allow to soak 4–8 hours and then drain.

2 Add the soaked chickpeas, 3 cups water, and salt to the inner pot. Secure the lid.

3 Press the Manual or Pressure Cook button and adjust the time to 10 minutes.

4 When the timer beeps, let pressure release naturally for 10 minutes, then quick-release any remaining pressure until float valve drops, then unlock lid.

5 Transfer the chickpeas to your food processor and add the avocado, oil, and lemon juice. Process until the mixture is super smooth. If the mixture is too thick, add water, 1 teaspoon at a time until desired consistency is reached.

6 Refrigerate until completely cooled and then sprinkle with crushed red pepper flakes and drizzle with the remaining ⅛ teaspoon olive oil before serving.

CALORIES: 129 | **FAT**: 7g | **PROTEIN**: 4g | **SODIUM**: 296mg
FIBER: 3g | **CARBOHYDRATES**: 14g | **SUGAR**: 2g

Avocado Deviled Eggs

Deviled eggs get a nutritional upgrade by adding avocado into the mix. Avocado is naturally creamy and mixes well with the other ingredients in this recipe. Be sure to find a mayonnaise that is made with avocado oil rather than an inflammatory oil like canola or soybean oil.

- **Hands-On Time: 15 minutes**
- **Cook Time: 7 minutes**

Serves 12

6 large eggs
1 medium avocado, peeled, pitted, and diced
2½ tablespoons mayonnaise
2 teaspoons lime juice
1 clove garlic, crushed
⅛ teaspoon cayenne pepper
⅛ teaspoon salt
1 medium jalapeño pepper, sliced
12 dashes hot sauce

PIPING BAG HACK

If you don't have a piping bag handy, cut off the end of a plastic sandwich bag and use that to pipe the filling into your egg whites.

1 Pour 1 cup water into the inner pot of your Instant Pot® and place the steam rack inside.

2 Carefully place the eggs directly onto the steam rack.

3 Press the Steam button and adjust the time to 7 minutes.

4 When the timer beeps, quick-release pressure until float valve drops and then unlock lid.

5 Immediately transfer the eggs to a bowl filled with iced water and let them sit 15 minutes.

6 Remove the eggs from the water and peel the shells away from the eggs. Slice the eggs in half.

7 Scoop egg yolks into a medium bowl and add the avocado, mayonnaise, lime juice, garlic, cayenne pepper, and salt.

8 Mash the egg yolk mixture until filling is evenly combined.

9 Spoon the filling into a piping bag and pipe filling into each egg white. Top each with a jalapeño slice and a dash of hot sauce.

CALORIES: 78 | **FAT**: 6g | **PROTEIN**: 3g | **SODIUM**: 68mg
FIBER: 1g | **CARBOHYDRATES**: 2g | **SUGAR**: 4g

Beans, Rice, and Whole Grains

The Instant Pot® will transform the way you think about cooking beans, rice, and whole grains. Traditionally it takes a good chunk of time and a lot of babysitting to cook these at home, but your Instant Pot® pressure cooker changes all that. Not only does it significantly reduce the cooking time, it also makes cooking beans, rice, and whole grains a mostly hands-off experience.

Many of the recipes in this chapter are perfect if you like to meal prep and prepare food for your week. Having a variety of cooked beans, rice, and whole grains in your refrigerator makes getting a healthy meal on the table much quicker and easier.

You'll notice the rice recipes call for stock as the cooking liquid. This is because of the flavor it adds to the final dish, but the same amount of water works just as well and you can season it after cooking.

Beans, rice, and whole grains are an important part of a well-rounded diet and provide a variety of nutrients your body needs. You will have fun exploring the recipes in this chapter, from lesser-known recipes such as Forbidden Rice to the basics everyone already loves like Basic Brown Rice and Black Beans.

Basic Brown Rice

This Basic Brown Rice recipe can be used as a side dish for a number of healthy meals, or as a meal-prep ingredient. The Instant Pot® gives you perfect rice every time, without having to constantly check to see if it's ready.

- **Hands-On Time: 1 minute**
- **Cook Time: 22 minutes**

Serves 4

1 cup brown rice
1 cup chicken stock

1 Place the rice and stock in the inner pot of the Instant Pot®. Secure the lid.

2 Press the Manual or Pressure Cook button and adjust the time to 22 minutes.

3 When the timer beeps, let pressure release naturally until float valve drops and then unlock lid.

4 Fluff the rice with a fork and serve.

CALORIES: 130 | **FAT**: 1g | **PROTEIN**: 4g | **SODIUM**: 86mg
FIBER: 2g | **CARBOHYDRATES**: 25g | **SUGAR**: 1g

Jasmine Rice

Jasmine rice has a delicate, floral scent and works well with a number of Asian dishes, especially Thai recipes. Jasmine rice can be used as a side dish for any meal that needs a quick starch.

- **Hands-On Time: 1 minute**
- **Cook Time: 3 minutes**

Serves 4

1 cup jasmine rice
1 cup water

1 Place the rice in a fine-mesh strainer and rinse it well.

2 Place the rice and water in the inner pot of the Instant Pot®. Secure the lid.

3 Press the Manual or Pressure Cook button and adjust the time to 3 minutes.

4 When the timer beeps, let pressure release naturally until float valve drops and then unlock lid.

5 Fluff the rice with a fork and serve.

CALORIES: 154 | **FAT**: 0g | **PROTEIN**: 3g | **SODIUM**: 1mg
FIBER: 0g | **CARBOHYDRATES**: 33g | **SUGAR**: 0g

Brown Rice with Lime and Cilantro

Simple brown rice is transformed with just a little lime and cilantro. It's amazing the way certain ingredients can totally elevate a dish—and that is the case with fresh lime juice and fresh cilantro. Those two ingredients make this a perfect companion for any Mexican or Tex-Mex–inspired meals you're creating in your kitchen.

- **Hands-On Time: 5 minutes**
- **Cook Time: 22 minutes**

Serves 4

1 cup brown rice

1 cup water

1 teaspoon salt

2 tablespoons extra-virgin olive oil

2 tablespoons fresh lime juice

1 cup chopped fresh cilantro

COMBINING RECIPES

A number of recipes in this book can be combined to create a complete meal. For this recipe, add Chili Lime Black Beans (see recipe in this chapter) and Steamed Broccoli (see recipe in Chapter 6) for a healthy and satisfying dinner.

1 Place the rice, water, and salt in the inner pot of the Instant Pot®. Secure the lid.

2 Press the Manual or Pressure Cook button and adjust the time to 22 minutes.

3 When the timer beeps, let pressure release naturally until float valve drops and then unlock lid.

4 Fluff the rice with a fork and transfer it to a large bowl. Allow the rice to cool for a few minutes and then add the olive oil, lime juice, and cilantro and gently stir to combine.

5 Serve.

CALORIES: 171 | **FAT**: 7g | **PROTEIN**: 2g | **SODIUM**: 583mg
FIBER: 2g | **CARBOHYDRATES**: 23g | **SUGAR**: 0g

Yellow Jasmine Rice

While jasmine rice is a rich source of B vitamins, here it gets a huge nutritional upgrade by adding fresh garlic and fresh turmeric. The result is a vibrantly hued yellow dish that is flavorful and nutritious. Both turmeric and garlic have been used medicinally for centuries and we are lucky that these two powerful foods also taste wonderful.

- **Hands-On Time: 5 minute**
- **Cook Time: 5 minutes**

Serves 4

1 cup jasmine rice
1 tablespoon avocado oil
2 cloves garlic, minced
1 tablespoon peeled and
    grated fresh turmeric
¼ teaspoon ground cumin
⅛ teaspoon ground cinnamon
1 cup chicken stock
½ cup chopped fresh cilantro

1 Place the rice in a fine-mesh strainer and rinse it well.

2 Press the Sauté button on the Instant Pot® and add the oil. Allow it to heat 1 minute and then add the garlic, turmeric, cumin, and cinnamon. Cook, stirring frequently, 1–2 minutes. Press the Cancel button.

3 Add the rice and stock and stir to combine. Use a spoon to scrape any brown bits that may be stuck to the bottom of the pot. Secure the lid.

4 Press the Manual or Pressure Cook button and adjust the time to 3 minutes.

5 When the timer beeps, let pressure release naturally until float valve drops and then unlock lid.

6 Fluff the rice with a fork and serve with fresh cilantro.

CALORIES: 216 | **FAT**: 4g | **PROTEIN**: 5g | **SODIUM**: 88mg
FIBER: 1g | **CARBOHYDRATES**: 38g | **SUGAR**: 1g

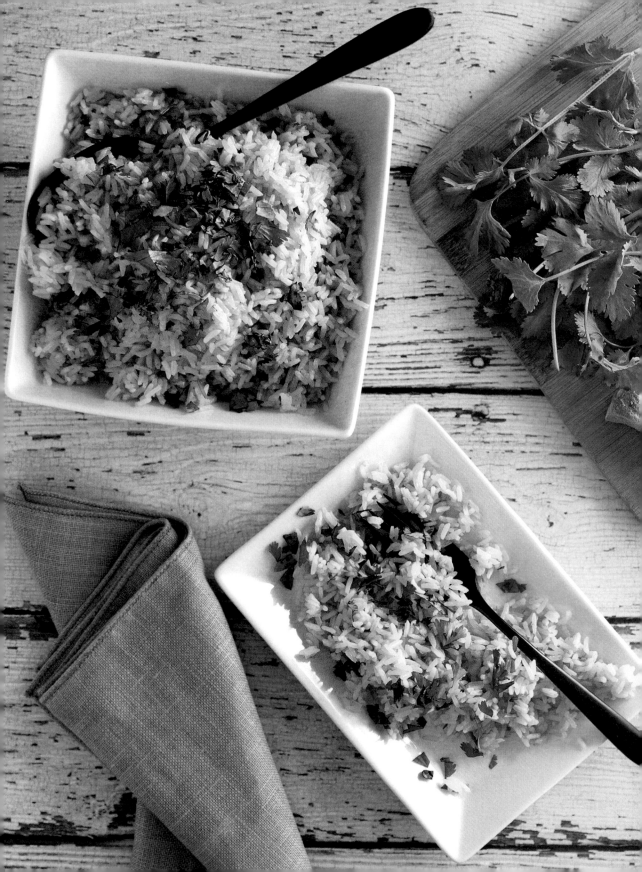

Wild Rice

Wild rice is higher in protein than most grains and it also is high in a number of vitamins and minerals. In addition, wild rice has a notably high concentration of antioxidants.

- **Hands-On Time: 1 minute**
- **Cook Time: 30 minutes**

Serves 4

1 cup wild rice
1 cup chicken stock

1 Place the rice and stock in the inner pot of the Instant Pot®. Secure the lid.

2 Press the Manual or Pressure Cook button and adjust the time to 30 minutes.

3 When the timer beeps, let pressure release naturally until float valve drops and then unlock lid.

4 Fluff the rice with a fork and serve.

CALORIES: 164 | **FAT**: 1g | **PROTEIN**: 7g | **SODIUM**: 88mg
FIBER: 2g | **CARBOHYDRATES**: 32g | **SUGAR**: 2g

Wild Rice Blend

This recipe makes a basic wild rice blend side dish that pairs perfectly with vegetables for a hearty vegetarian meal or is a perfect companion for your seafood dishes.

- **Hands-On Time: 1 minute**
- **Cook Time: 28 minutes**

Serves 4

1 cup wild rice blend
1 cup chicken stock

1 Place the rice and stock in the inner pot of the Instant Pot®. Secure the lid.

2 Press the Manual or Pressure Cook button and adjust the time to 28 minutes.

3 When the timer beeps, let pressure release naturally until float valve drops and then unlock lid.

4 Fluff the rice with a fork and serve.

CALORIES: 164 | **FAT**: 1g | **PROTEIN**: 7g | **SODIUM**: 88mg
FIBER: 2g | **CARBOHYDRATES**: 32g | **SUGAR**: 2g

Black Beans

You can save money by cooking your own black beans instead of buying them from a can, and the Instant Pot® makes it quicker and easier than ever. Soaking your beans ahead of time makes it even quicker and can also help with digestion. You can simply salt these beans and eat them as a side dish, or use this recipe for your meal prep and add them to a number of meals throughout your week.

- **Hands-On Time: 5 minutes**
- **Cook Time: 25 minutes**

Serves 8

1 pound dry black beans
6 cups water
2 teaspoons salt

1 Put the dry black beans in a bowl and cover with 3" water. Allow to soak 4–8 hours and then drain them.

2 Add the soaked black beans and 6 cups water to the inner pot. Secure the lid.

3 Press the Manual or Pressure Cook button and adjust the time to 25 minutes.

4 When the timer beeps, let pressure release naturally for 10 minutes, then quick-release any remaining pressure until float valve drops, then unlock lid.

5 Add the salt to the beans and then transfer to a bowl for serving or to an airtight container to store. These beans will keep in the refrigerator four to five days and can also be frozen up to six months.

CALORIES: 192 | FAT: 0g | PROTEIN: 12g | SODIUM: 586mg
FIBER: 9g | CARBOHYDRATES: 36g | SUGAR: 1g

Chili Lime Black Beans

Although you can make beans in the Instant Pot® without soaking them first, soaking them before cooking significantly reduces the cooking time. It's worth the extra effort to remember to place them in a bowl full of water the night before you plan to make this. You'll love the smoky flavor of these Chili Lime Black Beans. Don't skip the cilantro as it adds the perfect touch.

- **Hands-On Time: 5 minutes**
- **Cook Time: 10 minutes**

Serves 12

2 cups (1 pound) dry black
   beans
4 cups vegetable broth
1 tablespoon chili powder
1 teaspoon smoked paprika
¼ teaspoon salt
Juice from 1 large lime
½ cup chopped cilantro

HOW DO YOU LIKE YOUR BEANS?

The time it takes to cook your soaked beans can vary based on how firm you prefer your beans. Cooking 10 minutes will produce a cooked, yet firm bean that will hold up well. If you like a softer, mushier bean, add 5 minutes to the cooking time.

1 Place the beans in a large bowl and add enough water so the beans are covered by 3". Allow to soak at room temperature 4–8 hours.

2 Drain and rinse the beans. Place the beans, broth, chili powder, paprika, and salt in the inner pot and stir. Secure the lid.

3 Press the Manual or Pressure Cook button and adjust the time to 10 minutes.

4 When the timer beeps, let pressure release naturally until float valve drops and then unlock lid.

5 Stir in the lime juice and cilantro and serve.

CALORIES: 136 | FAT: 0g | PROTEIN: 8g | SODIUM: 251mg
FIBER: 7g | CARBOHYDRATES: 26g | SUGAR: 1g

Healthier Refried Beans

Refried beans are traditionally fried in lard or bacon grease. This recipe eliminates the unhealthy fats, but you're still getting plenty of flavor from the onion, garlic, and spices. The Instant Pot® makes it quicker and easier to make refried beans from scratch too! This makes a delicious side dish for a number of Mexican meals.

- **Hands-On Time: 11 minutes**
- **Cook Time: 27 minutes**

Serves 12

2 cups (1 pound) dry pinto beans
1 tablespoon avocado oil
1 large yellow onion, peeled and diced
4 cloves garlic, minced
7 cups water
2 teaspoons chili powder
1 teaspoon ground cumin
2 teaspoons salt

1 Place the beans in a large bowl and add enough water so the beans are covered by 2". Allow to soak at room temperature 4–8 hours.

2 Drain and rinse the beans.

3 Drizzle the oil in the Instant Pot®. Press the Sauté button and add the onion. Sauté the onion until it is softened and starting to brown, about 6 minutes.

4 Add the garlic and sauté an additional 30 seconds. Press the Cancel button.

5 Place the beans, water, chili powder, cumin, and salt into the inner pot. Secure the lid.

6 Press the Manual or Pressure Cook button and adjust the time to 20 minutes.

7 When the timer beeps, let pressure release naturally until float valve drops and then unlock lid.

8 Remove the lid and drain the beans, reserving the liquid. Place the drained beans back into the Instant Pot® and use an immersion blender or potato masher to blend or mash the beans to your desired consistency, adding in any of the reserved liquid as needed.

9 Transfer the beans to a bowl for serving. Refried beans may be stored in the refrigerator for three to four days or the freezer up to three months.

CALORIES: 149 | **FAT:** 2g | **PROTEIN:** 8g | **SODIUM:** 405mg
FIBER: 6g | **CARBOHYDRATES:** 25g | **SUGAR:** 1g

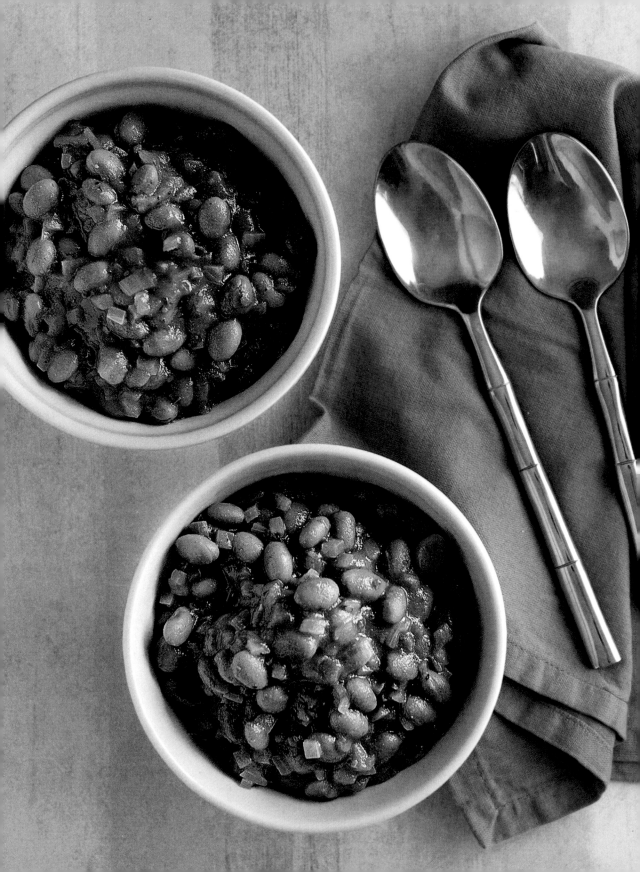

Saucy Pinto Beans

If you're looking for a perfect accompaniment for your Mexican dinner night, these Saucy Pinto Beans are the perfect pick. This bean dish is filled with bold flavors and will leave you satisfied. It is wonderful served with Basic Brown Rice (see recipe in this chapter) and a side vegetable for a complete meal.

- **Hands-On Time: 10 minutes**
- **Cook Time: 31 minutes**

Serves 8

2 cups (1 pound) dry pinto beans
2 tablespoons avocado oil
1 large yellow onion, peeled and diced
1 medium jalapeño, seeded and diced
2 teaspoons minced garlic
3½ cups chicken stock
1 (8-ounce) can tomato sauce
2 tablespoons chili powder
1 tablespoon yellow mustard
1 teaspoon dried oregano
1 teaspoon cumin
½ teaspoon black pepper
2 bay leaves
½ teaspoon salt

1 Place the beans in a bowl and cover with 3" water. Soak the beans 4–8 hours. Drain the beans.

2 Press the Sauté button of the Instant Pot® and add the oil. After the oil heats 1 minute add the onion, jalapeño, and garlic. Sauté until softened, about 5 minutes.

3 Add soaked beans, stock, tomato sauce, chili powder, mustard, oregano, cumin, pepper, bay leaves, and salt to the inner pot. Stir well to combine and scrape any brown bits from the bottom of the pot. Secure the lid.

4 Press the Manual or Pressure Cook button and adjust the time to 25 minutes.

5 When the timer beeps, let pressure release naturally until float valve drops and then unlock lid.

6 Remove and discard the bay leaves and then transfer the beans to a bowl for serving.

CALORIES: 289 | FAT: 5g | PROTEIN: 16g | SODIUM: 516mg
FIBER: 10g | CARBOHYDRATES: 44g | SUGAR: 5g

Tuscan White Beans

Cannelloni beans, or white kidney beans, are rich with both soluble and insoluble fiber. The fiber paired with iron, protein, folate, and copper make these beans a nutritional powerhouse you should include in your diet. This recipe makes it easy and inexpensive to do so, and the flavors are irresistible.

- **Hands-On Time: 5 minutes**
- **Cook Time: 28 minutes**

Serves 6

½ pound dry cannelloni beans

1 tablespoon avocado oil

3 large cloves garlic, smashed

¼ teaspoon crushed red pepper flakes

3 cups vegetable broth

1 Place the white beans in a large bowl and cover with 5 cups water. Soak the beans 4–8 hours.

2 Drain the soaked beans.

3 Press the Sauté button, add the oil, and allow to heat 2 minutes.

4 Add the garlic and red pepper flakes and let them sizzle for 30 seconds.

5 Add the beans and broth. Press the Cancel button. Secure the lid.

6 Press the Manual or Pressure Cook button and adjust the time to 25 minutes.

7 When the timer beeps, quick-release pressure until float valve drops and then unlock lid.

CALORIES: 156 | FAT: 3g | PROTEIN: 9g | SODIUM: 276mg
FIBER: 6g | CARBOHYDRATES: 25g | SUGAR: 1g

Spicy Black Beans

This is a dish that tastes much more indulgent than it is. Creamy and spicy, this black bean dish is always a big hit and makes enough to serve a crowd. The best part is that you can use dry black beans (such a money saver!) and they cook in 15 minutes.

- **Hands-On Time: 5 minutes**
- **Cook Time: 20 minutes**

Serves 6

½ pound dry black beans

1 (13.25-ounce) can unsweetened full-fat coconut milk

3 cups vegetable stock

1 tablespoon chopped fresh, peeled ginger

1 tablespoon red curry paste

½ teaspoon kosher salt

1 Place the beans in a large bowl and cover with 3" water. Soak the beans 4–8 hours. Drain the beans.

2 Place the soaked beans, coconut milk, stock, ginger, curry paste, and salt in the inner pot and stir until well combined. Secure the lid.

3 Press the Manual or Pressure Cook button and adjust the time to 20 minutes.

4 When the timer beeps, quick-release pressure until float valve drops and then unlock lid.

CALORIES: 263 | **FAT**: 13g | **PROTEIN**: 11g | **SODIUM**: 705mg
FIBER: 6g | **CARBOHYDRATES**: 27g | **SUGAR**: 1g

FORGET TO SOAK YOUR BEANS?

If you are ready to cook and forgot to soak your beans, it's okay! You can make this recipe with unsoaked beans; simply increase the cooking time to 25 minutes.

Forbidden Rice

Forbidden rice, also known as black rice, has a stunning purple-black color that will catch your eye. It gets its rich color from the anthocyanins it contains—the same class of antioxidants found in blueberries and blackberries.

- **Hands-On Time: 2 minutes**
- **Cook Time: 30 minutes**

Serves 4

1 cup forbidden rice
1 cup vegetable stock

1 Place the rice and stock in the inner pot of the Instant Pot®. Secure the lid.

2 Press the Manual or Pressure Cook button and adjust the time to 30 minutes.

3 When the timer beeps, let pressure release naturally until float valve drops and then unlock lid.

4 Fluff the rice with a fork and serve.

CALORIES: 114 | **FAT**: 1g | **PROTEIN**: 4g | **SODIUM**: 218mg
FIBER: 2g | **CARBOHYDRATES**: 22g | **SUGAR**: 1g

Teff

Teff is one of the lesser-known whole grains, but it is worth seeking out and giving it a try. Teff is a tiny grain that when cooked has a similar consistency to polenta. It has a light, sweet flavor and is a great source of fiber and protein. In addition, teff provides three times your recommended daily value of manganese. This is a health-promoting, gluten-free whole grain you should add to your dinner plate.

- **Hands-On Time: 1 minute**
- **Cook Time: 4 minutes**

Serves 4

1 cup dry teff
½ teaspoon salt
3 cups water

1 Add the teff, salt, and water to the inner pot. Secure the lid.

2 Press the Manual or Pressure Cook button and adjust the time to 4 minutes.

3 When the timer beeps, let pressure release naturally until float valve drops and then unlock lid.

CALORIES: 177 | **FAT**: 1g | **PROTEIN**: 6g | **SODIUM**: 296mg
FIBER: 4g | **CARBOHYDRATES**: 35g | **SUGAR**: 1g

Forbidden Rice with Lime, Mango, and Cilantro

The colors of this forbidden rice dish are stunning. The bright orange and greens contrast beautifully with the purple-black rice. This is a perfect dish to make ahead of time as that gives the flavors time to meld and that's when this dish is really spectacular.

- **Hands-On Time: 15 minutes**
- **Cook Time: 30 minutes**

Serves 4

1 cup forbidden rice

1 cup water

⅛ cup fresh lime juice

⅛ cup fresh orange juice

2 tablespoons extra-virgin olive oil

⅛ teaspoon salt

1 medium just-ripe mango, peeled, pitted, and cut into ½" dice

½ cup finely chopped red onion

½ cup unsalted almond slices

3 scallions, thinly sliced

1 medium jalapeño, seeded and minced

½ cup fresh cilantro leaves

1 Place the rice and water in the inner pot of the Instant Pot®. Secure the lid.

2 Press the Manual or Pressure Cook button and adjust the time to 30 minutes.

3 While the rice cooks, prepare the dressing. In a small bowl, add the lime juice, orange juice, oil, and salt and whisk well. Set aside.

4 When the timer beeps, let pressure release naturally until float valve drops and then unlock lid.

5 Fluff the rice with a fork and transfer to a medium bowl. Add the mango, onion, almond slices, scallions, and jalapeño and toss to combine. Add the dressing and cilantro and toss again to evenly coat. Serve cold or at room temperature.

CALORIES: 304 | **FAT**: 14g | **PROTEIN**: 7g | **SODIUM**: 79mg
FIBER: 5g | **CARBOHYDRATES**: 42g | **SUGAR**: 15g

Jasmine Rice with Mushrooms

Jasmine rice gets extra bulk and flavor with baby bella mushrooms. The Instant Pot® makes it simple, with everything cooking in one pot and enhancing the flavor at the same time. Speaking of flavor, the onion, garlic, and mushrooms make this a savory dish you'll crave over and over again. In addition to the incredible flavor mushrooms add to this dish, they also contain a powerful antioxidant, L-ergothioneine, which is known as a potent anti-inflammatory compound. It's a beautiful thing when amazing flavor and health benefits collide.

- **Hands-On Time: 5 minutes**
- **Cook Time: 15 minutes**

Serves 4

1 cup jasmine rice
1 tablespoon avocado oil
1 small yellow onion, peeled and chopped
10 ounces sliced baby bella mushrooms
3 cloves garlic, minced
¼ teaspoon salt
1 cup vegetable broth

1 Place the rice in a fine-mesh strainer and rinse well.

2 Press the Sauté button and add the oil to the inner pot. Allow it to heat 1 minute and then add the onion, mushrooms, garlic, and salt. Cook 5 minutes and then press the Cancel button.

3 Add the rice and broth and stir to combine. Secure the lid.

4 Press the Manual or Pressure Cook button and adjust the time to 10 minutes.

5 When the timer beeps, let pressure release naturally until float valve drops and then unlock lid.

6 Transfer to a bowl and serve immediately.

CALORIES: 229 | **FAT**: 4g | **PROTEIN**: 5g | **SODIUM**: 287mg
FIBER: 2g | **CARBOHYDRATES**: 43g | **SUGAR**: 2g

Basic Chickpeas

Chickpeas are a nutritious snack or addition to a variety of different meals. Add them to a salad for extra protein and fiber, as well as folate and manganese. Chickpeas also help keep blood sugar levels stable because they are considered a slow-releasing carbohydrate. This is an excellent recipe to use for meal prepping and it can save you money because it uses dry beans rather than canned.

- **Hands-On Time: 10 minutes**
- **Cook Time: 10 minutes**

Serves 8

2 cups (1 pound) dry chickpeas
6 cups water
2 teaspoons salt

1 Put the dry chickpeas in a large bowl and cover with 3" water. Allow to soak 4–8 hours and then drain.

2 Add the soaked chickpeas, 6 cups water, and salt to the inner pot. Secure the lid.

3 Press the Manual or Pressure Cook button and adjust the time to 10 minutes.

4 When the timer beeps, let pressure release naturally for 10 minutes, then quick-release any remaining pressure until float valve drops, then unlock lid.

5 Transfer to a bowl to serve or an airtight container to store. The chickpeas will keep in the refrigerator three to four days or in the freezer up to six months.

CALORIES: 214 | **FAT**: 3g | **PROTEIN**: 12g | **SODIUM**: 594mg
FIBER: 7g | **CARBOHYDRATES**: 36g | **SUGAR**: 6g

Spiced Millet

Millet is a quick-cooking whole grain that has a good amount of protein. It has a light, nutty flavor that is enhanced with warming spices in this dish. This recipe is perfect for any time you need a side dish to round out a meal. Add some chickpeas and steamed broccoli and it's a complete vegetarian meal.

- **Hands-On Time: 5 minutes**
- **Cook Time: 7 minutes**

Serves 6

1 tablespoon avocado oil

1 medium yellow onion, peeled and diced

¼ teaspoon ground cumin

¼ teaspoon ground cardamom

⅛ teaspoon ground cinnamon

1 bay leaf

2 cups millet

3 cups water

1 Press the Sauté button on the Instant Pot® and add the oil. Allow it to heat 1 minute, and then add the onion, cumin, cardamom, cinnamon, and bay leaf. Cook, stirring frequently, 5 minutes. Press the Cancel button.

2 Add the millet and water to the inner pot and stir to combine and scrape any brown bits that may be stuck to the bottom. Secure the lid.

3 Press the Manual or Pressure Cook button and adjust the time to 1 minute.

4 When the timer beeps, let pressure release naturally until float valve drops and then unlock lid.

5 Remove and discard the bay leaf and the transfer the millet to a bowl to serve.

CALORIES: 280 | FAT: 5g | PROTEIN: 8g | SODIUM: 4mg
FIBER: 6g | CARBOHYDRATES: 50g | SUGAR: 1g

Basic Quinoa

This recipe shows you how to make basic unflavored quinoa in your Instant Pot®. Once you are able to do this, you'll be able to use your cooked quinoa in a number of ways: as an addition to salad for extra protein and bulk, as part of a work lunch (just add some vegetables, chicken or beans, and a simple dressing), or even as a make-ahead breakfast dish that you can add almond milk and bananas to as you quickly reheat it in the morning.

- **Hands-On Time: 1 minute**
- **Cook Time: 1 minute**

Serves 4

1 cup dry quinoa
1 cup water

THE ANCIENT GRAIN THAT'S ACTUALLY A SEED
Quinoa is often called a grain, but in actuality, it's a seed. Even so, your body processes it much like other whole grains, so many people call it a pseudo cereal. Quinoa is rich in protein, fiber, B vitamins, and minerals.

1 Place the quinoa in a fine-mesh strainer and rinse under water until the water runs clear.

2 Add the quinoa and water to the inner pot. Secure the lid.

3 Press the Manual or Pressure Cook button and adjust the time to 1 minute.

4 When the timer beeps, let pressure release naturally until float valve drops and then unlock lid.

5 Fluff the quinoa with a fork and serve or store in an airtight container in the refrigerator.

CALORIES: 156 | **FAT**: 2g | **PROTEIN**: 6g | **SODIUM**: 2mg
FIBER: 3g | **CARBOHYDRATES**: 27g | **SUGAR**: 0g

White Bean Salad with Tomatoes and Avocado

When you need an easy and flavorful salad, turn to this White Bean Salad with Tomatoes and Avocado. The simple dressing doesn't overpower the star of the show: fresh basil. Fresh basil brings incredible flavor to this salad along with health benefits. Basil has compounds that inhibit the same pro-inflammatory cytokines as anti-inflammatory drugs! If you're lucky enough to have basil growing in your garden, you'll want to make this salad weekly. It's equally suitable as a light lunch as it is for a side dish you can bring to a potluck.

- **Hands-On Time: 10 minutes**
- **Cook Time: 25 minutes**

Serves 4

1 cup dry cannelloni beans

2 cups water

3 tablespoons extra-virgin olive oil

1 tablespoon lemon juice

1 clove garlic, minced

½ teaspoon coarse sea salt

¼ teaspoon black pepper

1 cup grape tomatoes, halved

1 large avocado, peeled, pitted, cut in half lengthwise, and sliced

1 cup packed basil leaves, chopped

MAKING THIS AHEAD OF TIME?

If you want to make this salad ahead of time, wait to add the avocado until just before serving. This will ensure you don't have brown avocado pieces.

1 Place the beans in a medium bowl and cover with 3" water. Soak the beans 4–8 hours. Drain the beans.

2 Place the beans and 2 cups water in the inner pot. Secure the lid.

3 Press the Manual or Pressure Cook button and adjust the time to 25 minutes.

4 Meanwhile, place the oil, lemon juice, garlic, salt, and pepper in a small container or jar with a tight lid. Shake until the ingredients are well combined; set aside.

5 When the timer beeps, let pressure release naturally until float valve drops and then unlock lid.

6 Allow the beans to cool, and then add them to a large bowl along with the tomatoes, avocado, and basil. Drizzle with the dressing and gently stir to coat.

CALORIES: 336 | **FAT:** 15g | **PROTEIN:** 13g | **SODIUM:** 205mg
FIBER: 16g | **CARBOHYDRATES:** 39g | **SUGAR:** 1g

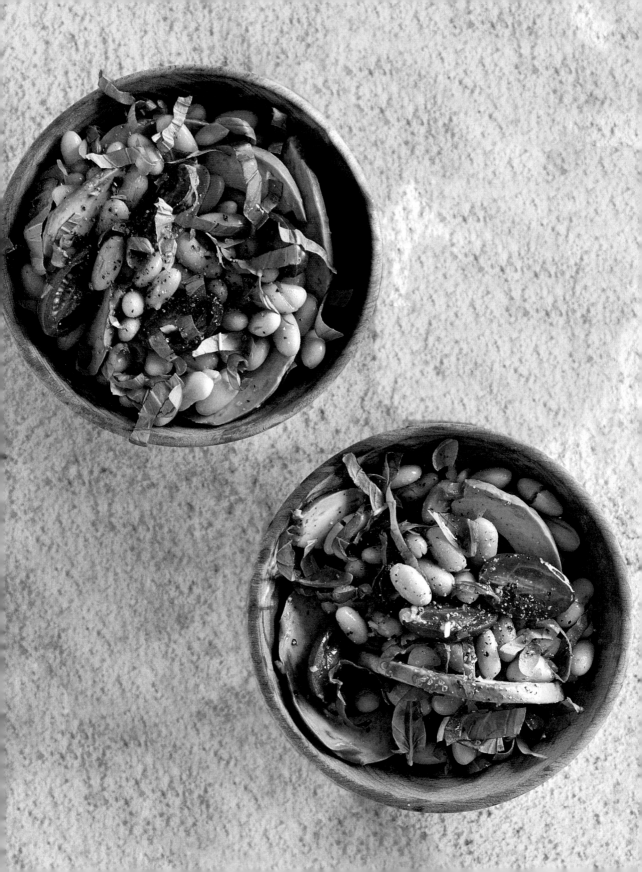

Creamy Tomato Lentils

Lentils aren't usually associated with tomatoes and Italian flavors, but after you try this dish, you'll wonder why it's not done more often. Even though coconut milk is used to make this dish creamy, you won't taste the coconut flavor.

- **Hands-On Time: 2 minutes**
- **Cook Time: 20 minutes**

Serves 6

1½ cups brown lentils

1 (15-ounce) can tomato sauce

2 tablespoons tomato paste

1 (15-ounce) can unsweetened full-fat coconut milk

⅓ cup water

1 teaspoon dried basil

1 teaspoon dried oregano

¼ teaspoon garlic salt

1 Place all of the ingredients in the inner pot and stir well to combine. Secure the lid.

2 Press the Manual or Pressure Cook button and adjust the time to 20 minutes.

3 When the timer beeps, let pressure release naturally until float valve drops and then unlock lid.

4 Stir and serve.

CALORIES: 330 | FAT: 15g | PROTEIN: 14g | SODIUM: 471mg
FIBER: 7g | CARBOHYDRATES: 37g | SUGAR: 4g

Coconut Curry Lentils

When dinnertime gets crazy, turn to this simple, flavorful dish that only requires you to dump the ingredients into your Instant Pot®.

- **Hands-On Time: 2 minutes**
- **Cook Time: 20 minutes**

Serves 6

1½ cups brown lentils

2 cups vegetable broth

2 tablespoons tomato paste

1 (15-ounce) can unsweetened full-fat coconut milk

2 teaspoons curry powder

½ teaspoon dried ginger

½ teaspoon dried oregano

¼ teaspoon garlic salt

1 Place all of the ingredients in the inner pot and stir well to combine. Secure the lid.

2 Press the Manual or Pressure Cook button and adjust the time to 20 minutes.

3 When the timer beeps, let pressure release naturally until float valve drops and then unlock lid.

4 Stir and serve.

CALORIES: 320 | FAT: 15g | PROTEIN: 14g | SODIUM: 316mg
FIBER: 6g | CARBOHYDRATES: 35g | SUGAR: 2g

6

Side Dishes

The side dishes in this chapter feature the planet's healthiest foods: vegetables. Consuming a wide variety of vegetables is the cornerstone of an anti-inflammatory diet. Vegetables are filled with phytonutrients that work in your body to build your immune system and fight inflammation. The more vegetables you fill your plate with, the more likely your body is to have a healthy inflammatory response and the healthier you will be in the long run.

While this chapter is filled with vegetable dishes that are considered side dishes, that doesn't mean they aren't the star of the meal. The healthiest people in the world ensure that vegetables make up the bulk of their diet. Vegetables can be easy to prepare and delicious, and thankfully, the Instant Pot® makes it quick to get those vegetables from your refrigerator onto your dinner plate.

Adding a number of "side dishes" to your plate is an excellent way to construct a complete meal. Consider mixing and matching the recipes in this chapter with the recipes in the Beans, Rice, and Whole Grains chapter to create hearty and delicious vegan meals.

Enjoy the fresh bounty of vegetables with the recipes in this chapter!

Steamed Broccoli

Broccoli is packed with vitamins, minerals, and potent antioxidants that all contribute to overall health. This recipe pairs so well with the Vegetable "Cheese" Sauce (see recipe in this chapter).

- **Hands-On Time: 5 minutes**
- **Cook Time: 1 minute**

Serves 6

6 cups broccoli florets

1 Pour 1½ cups water into the inner pot of the Instant Pot®. Place a steam rack inside.

2 Place the broccoli florets inside a steamer basket and place the basket on the steam rack.

3 Press the Steam button and adjust the time to 1 minute.

4 When the timer beeps, quick-release pressure until float valve drops and then unlock lid.

5 Remove the steamer basket and serve.

CALORIES: 30 | **FAT**: 0g | **PROTEIN**: 3g | **SODIUM**: 30mg
FIBER: 2g | **CARBOHYDRATES**: 6g | **SUGAR**: 2g

Boiled Cabbage

Cabbage is loaded with flavonoids that have strong anti-inflammatory benefits and are also known to have anticancer properties. This cabbage dish is anything but basic despite its simple ingredient list.

- **Hands-On Time: 5 minutes**
- **Cook Time: 5 minutes**

Serves 6

1 large head green cabbage, cored and chopped
3 cups vegetable broth
1 teaspoon salt
½ teaspoon black pepper

1 Place the cabbage, broth, salt, and pepper in the inner pot. Secure the lid.

2 Press the Manual or Pressure Cook button and adjust the time to 5 minutes.

3 When the timer beeps, quick-release pressure until float valve drops and then unlock lid.

4 Serve the cabbage with a little of the cooking liquid.

CALORIES: 54 | **FAT**: 0g | **PROTEIN**: 3g | **SODIUM**: 321mg
FIBER: 5g | **CARBOHYDRATES**: 13g | **SUGAR**: 7g

Vegetable "Cheese" Sauce

If you are a person who just can't find a love of vegetables without a little something extra, this is the recipe you need. Instead of a dairy-filled sauce that causes inflammation, though, here's a creamy, cheese-flavored sauce that actually has incredible nutrition all on its own because it's made with vegetables! This is a great sauce for steamed broccoli, cauliflower, and more.

- **Hands-On Time: 15 minutes**
- **Cook Time: 11 minutes**

Serves 6

1 small yellow onion, peeled and chopped

1 medium zucchini, peeled and sliced

6 cloves garlic, chopped

2¼ cups vegetable broth, divided

¼ teaspoon paprika

1 medium sweet potato, peeled and chopped

½ cup nutritional yeast

1 Place the onion, zucchini, garlic, and ¼ cup broth into the inner pot. Press the Sauté button and let the vegetables sauté until soft, 5 minutes. Press the Cancel button.

2 Add the remaining 2 cups broth, paprika, and sweet potato. Secure the lid.

3 Press the Manual or Pressure Cook button and adjust the time to 6 minutes.

4 When the timer beeps, quick-release pressure until float valve drops and then unlock lid.

5 Allow to cool for a few minutes and then transfer the mixture to a large blender.

6 Add the nutritional yeast to the blender with the other ingredients and blend on high until thoroughly combined and smooth.

7 Serve warm as a topping for the vegetables of your choice.

CALORIES: 58 | FAT: 0g | PROTEIN: 4g | SODIUM: 226mg
FIBER: 3g | CARBOHYDRATES: 10g | SUGAR: 3g

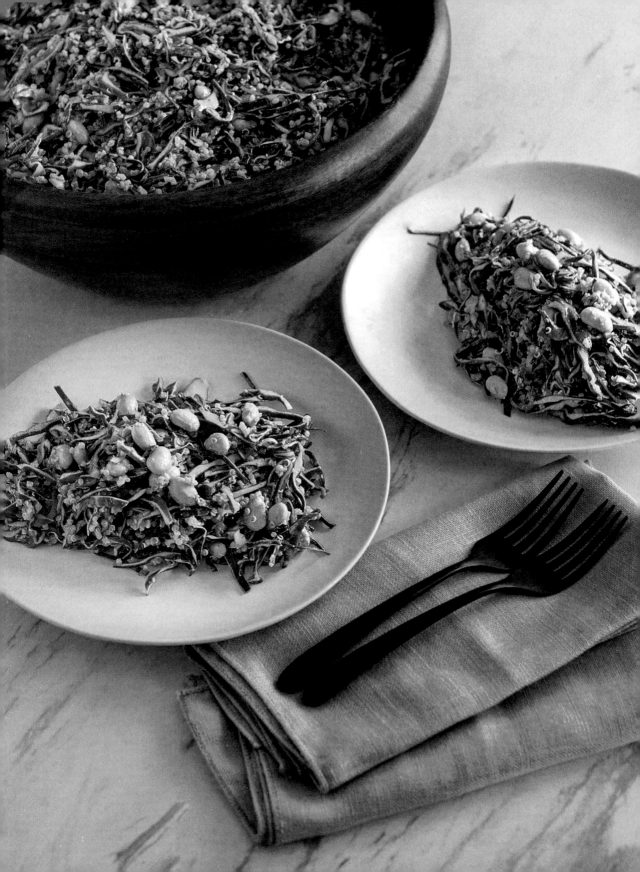

Purple Cabbage Salad with Quinoa and Edamame

This cabbage dish has Asian-inspired flavor and could not be easier to put together. While the quinoa and edamame are cooking, chop your cabbage and make your dressing. Then it comes together quickly for a hearty, satisfying, and flavorful side dish. Embrace the beautiful color of purple cabbage knowing those deep hues signify powerful antioxidants.

- **Hands-On Time: 7 minutes**
- **Cook Time: 2 minutes**

Serves 8

½ cup dry quinoa

1 (10-ounce) bag frozen shelled edamame

1 cup vegetable broth

¼ cup reduced sodium tamari

¼ cup natural almond butter

3 tablespoons toasted sesame seed oil

½ teaspoon pure stevia powder

1 head purple cabbage, cored and chopped

EAT THE RAINBOW

The bright, beautiful color you find in purple cabbage is a strong indicator of its nutritional content. Remember that eating the full spectrum of colors of foods is one of the most important parts of eating an anti-inflammatory diet.

1 Place the quinoa, edamame, and broth in the inner pot of your Instant Pot® and secure the lid. Press the Manual or Pressure Cook button and adjust the time to 2 minutes.

2 Meanwhile, in a small bowl, whisk together the tamari, almond butter, sesame seed oil, and stevia. Set aside.

3 When the timer beeps, quick-release pressure until float valve drops and then unlock lid.

4 Use a fork to fluff the quinoa, and then transfer the mixture to a large bowl. Allow the quinoa and edamame to cool, and then add the purple cabbage to the bowl and toss to combine.

5 Add the dressing and toss again until everything is evenly coated. Serve.

CALORIES: 220 | **FAT**: 11g | **PROTEIN**: 10g | **SODIUM**: 313mg
FIBER: 7g | **CARBOHYDRATES**: 21g | **SUGAR**: 5g

Steamed Cauliflower

Cauliflower is used in so many ways these days. Want a gluten-free pizza crust? Cauliflower. Want low-carb rice? Cauliflower. Sometimes, though, it's nice to just enjoy this nutritious and versatile vegetable for what it is. Cauliflower, plain and simple. Cauliflower is an excellent source of antioxidants, which protects your body from harmful free radicals and inflammation. It's worth adding to your dinner plate! Eat this dish alone or pair it with the Vegetable "Cheese" Sauce in this chapter.

- **Hands-On Time: 5 minutes**
- **Cook Time: 2 minutes**

Serves 6

1 large head cauliflower, cored and cut into large florets

ANOTHER USE FOR STEAMED CAULIFLOWER

Chill the steamed cauliflower in your refrigerator and then try it in your breakfast smoothie. It makes a creamy addition and boosts the nutrition!

1 Pour 2 cups water into the inner pot of the Instant Pot®. Place a steam rack inside.

2 Place the cauliflower florets inside a steamer basket and place the basket on the steam rack.

3 Press the Steam button and adjust the time to 2 minutes.

4 When the timer beeps, quick-release pressure until float valve drops and then unlock lid.

5 Carefully remove the steamer basket and serve.

CALORIES: 34 | FAT: 0g | PROTEIN: 3g | SODIUM: 41mg
FIBER: 3g | CARBOHYDRATES: 7g | SUGAR: 3g

Saucy Brussels Sprouts and Carrots

If you've ever thought vegetables are tasteless, bland, or boring, this is the recipe you need to try. Brussels sprouts and carrots swim in a dreamy sauce that will awaken your taste buds and put to rest any hesitations you have. Serve this dish with brown rice to soak up the tasty sauce and you have yourself a vegan meal. Research shows that eating more vegetarian meals can lower the serum levels of C-reactive protein, which is a biomarker of inflammation. It would be equally delicious with a simple chicken breast on the side and the sauce can do double duty!

- **Hands-On Time: 15 minutes**
- **Cook Time: 12 minutes**

Serves 4

1 tablespoon coconut oil

12 ounces Brussels sprouts, tough ends removed and cut in half

12 ounces carrots (about 4 medium), peeled, ends removed, and cut into 1" chunks

¼ cup fresh lime juice

¼ cup apple cider vinegar

½ cup coconut aminos

¼ cup almond butter

1 Press the Sauté button and melt the oil in the inner pot. Add the Brussels sprouts and carrots and sauté until browned, about 5–7 minutes.

2 While the vegetables are browning, make the sauce. In a small bowl, whisk together the lime juice, vinegar, coconut aminos, and almond butter.

3 Pour the sauce over the vegetables and press the Cancel button. Secure the lid.

4 Press the Manual or Pressure Cook button and adjust the time to 6 minutes.

5 When the timer beeps, quick-release pressure until float valve drops and then unlock lid.

CALORIES: 216 | **FAT**: 11g | **PROTEIN**: 6g | **SODIUM**: 738mg
FIBER: 6g | **CARBOHYDRATES**: 22g | **SUGAR**: 5g

THE SCOOP ON COCONUT AMINOS

Coconut aminos is a sauce that has a flavor similar to soy sauce, but it's from the sap of the coconut. It's sweeter than soy sauce, but has similar qualities in that it's dark, deeply flavored, and salty. Because it is soy- and gluten-free, it's an excellent substitute for those avoiding soy and gluten.

Simple Spaghetti Squash

Spaghetti squash gets its name from its long spaghetti-like strands that you can twirl around your fork as if you were eating pasta. Although its taste and texture isn't exactly like pasta, it can be a good stand-in. Spaghetti squash is high in vitamins A and C, two nutrients that help prevent free radical damage and inflammation. This is a basic spaghetti squash recipe, simply dressed with olive oil and seasoned with salt and pepper. Sometimes simple is best, because you'll find yourself craving this simple side dish at every meal!

- **Hands-On Time: 2 minutes**
- **Cook Time: 25 minutes**

Serves 4

1 medium spaghetti squash
2 tablespoons extra virgin olive oil
⅛ teaspoon salt
⅛ teaspoon black pepper

1 Place 1½ cups water in the inner pot of your Instant Pot®. Place the steam rack inside.

2 Wash squash with soap and water and dry it. Place the whole uncut squash on top of the steam rack inside the inner pot. Secure the lid.

3 Press the Manual or Pressure Cook button and adjust the time to 25 minutes.

4 When the timer beeps, quick-release pressure until float valve drops and then unlock lid.

5 Allow the squash to cool, and then carefully remove it from the pot. Use a sharp knife to cut the squash in half lengthwise. Spoon out the seeds and discard. Use a fork to scrape out the squash strands into a medium bowl.

6 Drizzle with the oil, add the salt and pepper, and serve.

CALORIES: 122 | **FAT**: 7g | **PROTEIN**: 2g | **SODIUM**: 114mg
FIBER: 3g | **CARBOHYDRATES**: 15g | **SUGAR**: 6g

Perfect "Baked" Sweet Potatoes

Baked sweet potatoes make an excellent side dish to round out so many meals, but they take an entire hour to bake in the oven. The Instant Pot® comes to the rescue again, allowing you to have "baked" sweet potatoes even on weeknights. This recipe calls for topping them simply with coconut oil and cinnamon, but there's room to get creative and top them however you prefer. Whatever you decide, include sweet potatoes in your diet often. Their bright, vibrant orange color is indicative of the presence of potent antioxidants that fight inflammation!

- **Hands-On Time: 2 minutes**
- **Cook Time: 18 minutes**

Serves 4

4 medium sweet potatoes
2 tablespoons coconut oil
½ teaspoon ground cinnamon

1 Pour 1½ cups water into the Instant Pot® and place the steam rack inside.

2 Place the sweet potatoes on the rack. It's okay if they overlap. Secure the lid.

3 Press the Manual or Pressure Cook button and adjust the time to 18 minutes.

4 When the timer beeps, quick-release pressure until float valve drops and then unlock lid.

5 Carefully remove the sweet potatoes from the pot. Use a knife to cut each sweet potato lengthwise and open the potato slightly. Add ½ tablespoon coconut oil and ⅛ teaspoon cinnamon to each potato and serve.

CALORIES: 171 | FAT: 6g | PROTEIN: 2g | SODIUM: 71mg
FIBER: 4g | CARBOHYDRATES: 26g | SUGAR: 5g

Lemony Cauliflower Rice

For those times when you want extra vegetables with your dinner instead of rice, you can turn to cauliflower rice. Riced cauliflower is made from cauliflower that's been chopped finely or processed in a food processor. If you use your food processor, make sure to not overprocess or you'll end up with mushy cauliflower rice. You're going to love the rice-like texture and lemony texture of this cauliflower rice dish. Cauliflower is a rich source of vitamin C, which is known to help control chronic inflammation.

- **Hands-On Time: 10 minutes**
- **Cook Time: 8 minutes**

Serves 4

1 tablespoon avocado oil
1 small yellow onion, peeled and diced
1 teaspoon minced garlic
4 cups riced cauliflower
Juice from 1 small lemon
½ teaspoon salt
¼ teaspoon black pepper

TIME-SAVING TIP
Instead of buying a head of cauliflower and turning it into riced cauliflower yourself, you can save time by purchasing cauliflower that's already been riced for you. Most supermarkets carry riced cauliflower in the produce section or the frozen vegetables section.

1 Press the Sauté button, add the oil to the pot, and heat 1 minute.

2 Add the onion and sauté 5 minutes.

3 Add the garlic and sauté 1 more minute. Press the Cancel button.

4 Add the cauliflower rice, lemon juice, salt, and pepper and stir to combine. Secure the lid.

5 Press the Manual or Pressure Cook button and adjust the time to 1 minute.

6 When the timer beeps, quick-release pressure until float valve drops and then unlock lid.

7 Transfer to a bowl for serving.

CALORIES: 60 | FAT: 3g | PROTEIN: 2g | SODIUM: 311mg
FIBER: 2g | CARBOHYDRATES: 6g | SUGAR: 3g

Lemony Steamed Asparagus

Look for thick asparagus as the thin spears will cook too quickly. Both asparagus and lemon juice are high in anti-inflammatory nutrients, making this a potent combination!

- **Hands-On Time: 5 minutes**
- **Cook Time: 0 minutes**

Serves 4

1 pound asparagus, woody ends removed
Juice from ½ large lemon
¼ teaspoon kosher salt

1 Add ½ cup water to the inner pot and add the steam rack. Add the asparagus to the steamer basket and place the basket on top of the rack.

2 Press the Steam button and adjust the time to 0 minutes.

3 When the timer beeps, quick-release pressure until float valve drops and then unlock lid.

4 Transfer the asparagus to a plate and top with lemon juice and salt.

CALORIES: 13 | **FAT**: 0g | **PROTEIN**: 1g | **SODIUM**: 146mg
FIBER: 1g | **CARBOHYDRATES**: 3g | **SUGAR**: 1g

Lemon Garlic Red Chard

The dark green leaves and deep red stems of red chard indicate the presence of strong phytonutrients and antioxidants that help your body have a positive inflammatory response.

- **Hands-On Time: 10 minutes**
- **Cook Time: 7 minutes**

Serves 4

1 tablespoon avocado oil
1 small yellow onion, peeled and diced
1 bunch red chard, leaves and stems chopped and kept separate (about 12 ounces)
3 cloves garlic, minced
¾ teaspoon salt
Juice from ½ medium lemon
1 teaspoon lemon zest

1 Add the oil to the inner pot of the Instant Pot® and allow it to heat 1 minute. Add the onion and chard stems and sauté 5 minutes. Add the garlic and sauté another 30 seconds. Add the chard leaves, salt, and lemon juice and stir to combine. Press the Cancel button. Secure the lid.

2 Press the Manual or Pressure Cook button and adjust the time to 0 minutes.

3 When the timer beeps, quick-release pressure until float valve drops and then unlock lid.

4 Spoon the chard mixture into a serving bowl and top with lemon zest.

CALORIES: 57 | **FAT**: 3g | **PROTEIN**: 2g | **SODIUM**: 617mg
FIBER: 2g | **CARBOHYDRATES**: 6g | **SUGAR**: 2g

Lemon Ginger Broccoli and Carrots

Fresh ginger gives a zesty bite to two familiar vegetables. Not only is fresh ginger a great flavor enhancer for many dishes, it also adds its strong anti-inflammatory powers. It's been used medicinally for centuries and is helpful to incorporate into your diet as often as possible. It's a perfect match with fresh garlic to flavor the carrots and broccoli in this recipe.

- **Hands-On Time: 10 minutes**
- **Cook Time: 5 minutes**

Serves 6

1 tablespoon avocado oil

1" fresh ginger, peeled and thinly sliced

1 clove garlic, minced

2 broccoli crowns, stems removed and cut into large florets

2 large carrots, peeled and thinly sliced

½ teaspoon kosher salt

Juice from ½ large lemon

¼ cup water

1 Add the oil to the inner pot. Press the Sauté button and heat oil 2 minutes.

2 Add the ginger and garlic and sauté 1 minute. Add the broccoli, carrots, and salt and stir to combine. Press the Cancel button.

3 Add the lemon juice and water and use a wooden spoon to scrape up any brown bits. Secure the lid.

4 Press the Manual or Pressure Cook button and adjust the time to 2 minutes.

5 When the timer beeps, quick-release pressure until float valve drops and then unlock lid.

6 Serve immediately.

CALORIES: 67 | FAT: 2g | PROTEIN: 3g | SODIUM: 245mg
FIBER: 3g | CARBOHYDRATES: 10g | SUGAR: 3g

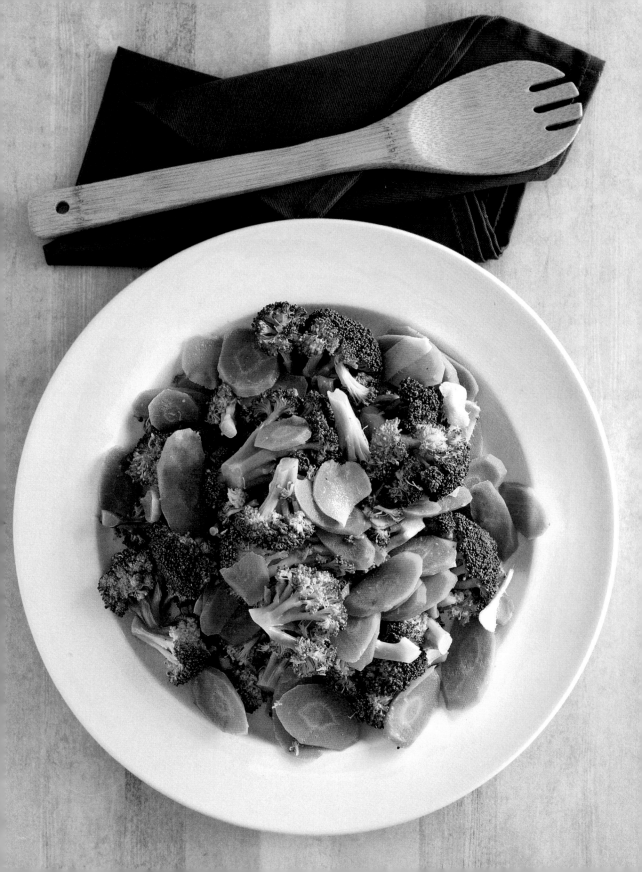

Wilted Spinach Salad with Quinoa

If you've never experienced a warm spinach salad, you're in for a treat with this recipe. Quinoa and vegetables are cooked to perfection in the Instant Pot®, and then while still warm, tossed with raw baby spinach leaves. After being drizzled with a light dressing, the whole thing is tossed together, wilting the leaves just a touch. Heating the spinach leaves makes a warm, satisfying salad, but it also allows for better absorption of the rich inflammation-fighting nutrients with which spinach is filled! Add some chopped hard-boiled eggs to make this a hearty vegetarian salad that is a meal all in itself.

- **Hands-On Time: 15 minutes**
- **Cook Time: 7 minutes**

Serves 6

¼ cup extra-virgin olive oil

2 tablespoons fresh lemon juice

¼ teaspoon pure stevia powder

1 teaspoon Dijon mustard

¼ teaspoon salt

⅛ teaspoon black pepper

1 tablespoon avocado oil

1 small yellow onion, peeled and diced

1 large carrot, peeled and diced

1 medium stalk celery, ends removed and sliced

½ cup dry quinoa

1 cup vegetable broth

10 ounces baby spinach leaves

1 In a small bowl, whisk together the olive oil, lemon juice, stevia, mustard, salt, and pepper. Set aside.

2 Add the avocado oil to the inner pot of the Instant Pot® and press the Sauté button. Allow the oil to heat 1 minute and then add the onion, carrot, and celery. Cook the vegetables until they are softened, about 5 minutes.

3 Rinse the quinoa in a fine-mesh strainer under water until the water runs clear. Add the quinoa to the inner pot and stir to combine with the vegetables. Press the Cancel button.

4 Add the vegetable broth to the inner pot and secure the lid. Press the Manual or Pressure Cook button and adjust the time to 1 minute.

5 When the timer beeps, quick-release pressure until float valve drops and then unlock lid.

6 Place the spinach leaves in a large bowl and top with the quinoa mixture. Drizzle with the dressing and toss to combine. Serve warm.

CALORIES: 178 | **FAT**: 12g | **PROTEIN**: 4g | **SODIUM**: 259mg
FIBER: 3g | **CARBOHYDRATES**: 14g | **SUGAR**: 2g

Curried Mustard Greens

One of the best things you can do for yourself if you're eating an anti-inflammatory diet is to eat a wide variety of green vegetables, especially leafy greens. This flavorful dish is the perfect way to add a not-so-common green to your diet. You can adjust the heat of this recipe by using a mild or spicy curry powder.

- **Hands-On Time: 15 minutes**
- **Cook Time: 10 minutes**

Serves 6

1 tablespoon avocado oil

1 medium white onion, peeled and chopped

1 tablespoon peeled and chopped ginger

3 cloves garlic, minced

2 tablespoons curry powder

½ teaspoon salt

¼ teaspoon black pepper

2 cups vegetable broth

½ cup coconut cream

1 large bunch mustard greens (about 1 pound), tough stems removed and roughly chopped

1 Add the oil to the inner pot. Press the Sauté button and heat the oil 2 minutes.

2 Add the onion and sauté until softened, about 5 minutes.

3 Add the ginger, garlic, curry, salt, and pepper and sauté 1 more minute.

4 Stir in the vegetable broth and coconut cream until combined and then allow it to come to a boil, about 2–3 minutes more. Press the Cancel button.

5 Stir in the mustard greens until everything is well combined. Secure the lid.

6 Press the Manual or Pressure Cook button and adjust the time to 0 minutes.

7 When the timer beeps, quick-release pressure until float valve drops and then unlock lid.

8 Transfer to a bowl and serve.

CALORIES: 124 | **FAT**: 9g | **PROTEIN**: 3g | **SODIUM**: 388mg
FIBER: 4g | **CARBOHYDRATES**: 9g | **SUGAR**: 2g

"Cheesy" Brussels Sprouts and Carrots

These Brussels sprouts and carrots taste so indulgent with the "cheesy" sauce, but in reality are packed with nutrition.

- **Hands-On Time: 10 minutes**
- **Cook Time: 10 minutes**

Serves 4

1 pound Brussels sprouts, tough ends removed and cut in half
1 pound baby carrots
1 cup chicken stock
2 tablespoons lemon juice
½ cup nutritional yeast
¼ teaspoon salt

1 Add the Brussels sprouts, carrots, stock, lemon juice, nutritional yeast, and salt to the inner pot of your Instant Pot®. Stir well to combine. Secure the lid.

2 Press the Manual or Pressure Cook button and adjust the time to 10 minutes.

3 When the timer beeps, quick-release pressure until float valve drops and then unlock lid. Transfer the vegetables and sauce to a bowl and serve.

CALORIES: 134 | **FAT**: 1g | **PROTEIN**: 9g | **SODIUM**: 340mg
FIBER: 8g | **CARBOHYDRATES**: 23g | **SUGAR**: 8g

Garlic Green Beans

Green beans make a quick and easy side dish that goes with almost any meal and the Instant Pot® cooks them to crisp tender perfection.

- **Hands-On Time: 2 minutes**
- **Cook Time: 5 minutes**

Serves 4

12 ounces green beans, ends trimmed
4 cloves garlic, minced
1 tablespoon avocado oil
½ teaspoon salt
1 cup water

1 Place the green beans in a medium bowl and toss with the garlic, oil, and salt. Transfer this mixture to the steamer basket.

2 Pour 1 cup water into the inner pot and place the steam rack inside. Place the steamer basket with the green beans on top of the steam rack. Secure the lid.

3 Press the Manual or Pressure Cook button and adjust the time to 5 minutes.

4 When the timer beeps, quick-release pressure until float valve drops and then unlock lid.

5 Transfer to a bowl for serving.

CALORIES: 58 | **FAT**: 3g | **PROTEIN**: 2g | **SODIUM**: 295mg
FIBER: 2g | **CARBOHYDRATES**: 6g | **SUGAR**: 2g

Simple Beet Salad

If you have bad memories of beets from your childhood, try to open your mind and give them another chance. In this salad they are dressed with a flavorful dressing and combined with the crunch of raw celery, and they'll make you realize there's so much more to beets than the bland canned variety your parents served you. The vibrant color of beets is thanks to the pigments they contain, known as betalains, and it's what gives them their powerful anti-inflammatory powers!

- **Hands-On Time: 15 minutes**
- **Cook Time: 5 minutes**

Serves 8

6 medium beets, peeled and
   cut into small cubes
1 cup water
¼ cup extra-virgin olive oil
¼ cup apple cider vinegar
1 teaspoon Dijon mustard
¼ teaspoon pure stevia
   powder
½ teaspoon salt
¼ teaspoon black pepper
1 large shallot, peeled and
   diced
1 large stalk celery, ends
   removed and thinly sliced

1 Place the beets into the steamer basket.

2 Pour 1 cup water into the inner pot and place the steam rack inside. Place the steamer basket with the beets on top of the steam rack.

3 Meanwhile, in a small container or jar with a tight lid add the oil, vinegar, mustard, stevia, salt, and pepper and shake well to combine. Set aside. Secure the lid.

4 Press the Manual or Pressure Cook button and adjust the time to 5 minutes.

5 When the timer beeps, quick-release pressure until float valve drops and then unlock lid.

6 Carefully remove the basket from the Instant Pot® and let the beets cool completely.

7 Place the shallot and celery in a large bowl and then add the cooked, cooled beets. Drizzle with the dressing and toss to coat.

CALORIES: 91 | **FAT**: 7g | **PROTEIN**: 1g | **SODIUM**: 215mg
FIBER: 2g | **CARBOHYDRATES**: 7g | **SUGAR**: 4g

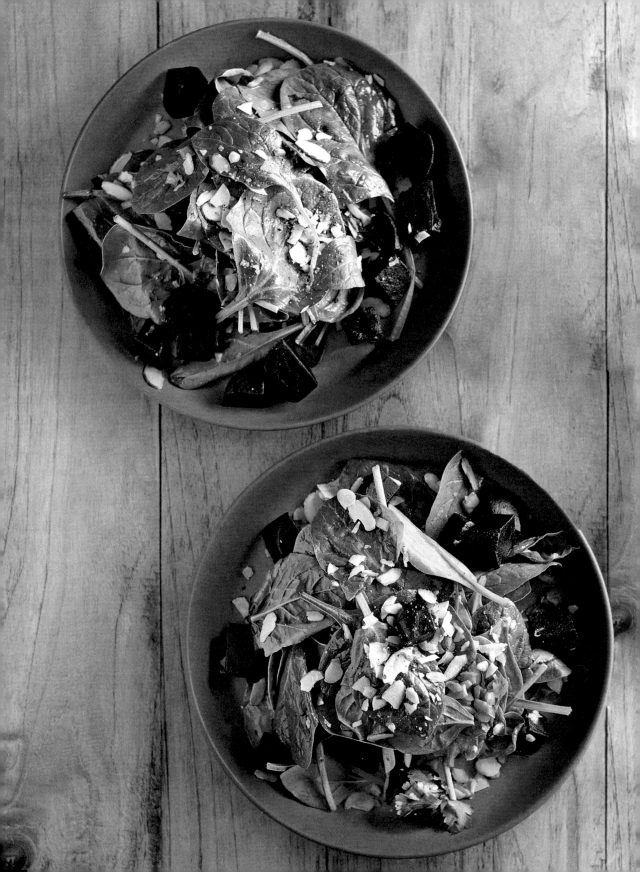

Spinach Salad with Beets, Almonds, and Citrus Vinaigrette

Beets have powerful antioxidants called betalains that are known for their anti-inflammatory and detoxifying properties. This recipe is one of the easiest (and tastiest!) ways to enjoy cooked beets. Beets have an earthy flavor that is offset by a sweet citrus vinaigrette in this bright and flavorful salad. You can add the beets to the salad warm or wait for them to cool, either way they complement this nutritious salad perfectly.

- **Hands-On Time: 7 minutes**
- **Cook Time: 5 minutes**

Serves 4

3 medium beets, peeled and cut into small cubes

1 cup water

½ small shallot, peeled and finely chopped

⅓ cup extra-virgin olive oil

2 tablespoons apple cider vinegar

2½ tablespoons fresh orange juice

¼ teaspoon orange zest

5 ounces baby spinach leaves

¼ cup sliced almonds

⅛ teaspoon coarse salt

⅛ teaspoon freshly ground black pepper

1 Place the beets into the steamer basket.

2 Pour 1 cup water into the inner pot and place the steam rack inside. Place the steamer basket with the beets on top of the steam rack.

3 Meanwhile, in a container or jar with a tight lid add the shallot, oil, vinegar, orange juice, and orange zest and shake well to combine. Set aside. Secure the lid.

4 Press the Manual or Pressure Cook button and adjust the time to 5 minutes.

5 When the timer beeps, quick-release pressure until float valve drops and then unlock lid.

6 Place the spinach and almonds in a large bowl and add the cooked beets. Drizzle with the dressing and toss to coat. Top the salad with salt and pepper and serve.

CALORIES: 234 | **FAT**: 20g | **PROTEIN**: 3g | **SODIUM**: 125mg
FIBER: 3g | **CARBOHYDRATES**: 10g | **SUGAR**: 6g

Herbed Mashed Sweet Potatoes

The Instant Pot® transforms sweet potatoes, normally a hard, dense vegetable, into something soft, tender, and easy to mash. Adding extra-virgin olive oil when you're mashing helps coat the starch particles of the spud and yields a creamy, not gluey result. The herbs add a savory flavor that balances the natural sweetness of the orange-hued potatoes.

- **Hands-On Time: 10 minutes**
- **Cook Time: 8 minutes**

Serves 6

1 cup water
3 large sweet potatoes, peeled and cut into cubes
2 tablespoons extra virgin olive oil
1 teaspoon dried thyme
1 teaspoon dried rosemary, crushed
¼ teaspoon garlic salt

SWEET POTATOES OR YAMS?

There are many different varieties of sweet potatoes, ranging in color from white to orange to purple. The sweet, orange-hued potato is what is recommended for this recipe. Even though many times this type of sweet potato is mistakenly called a yam, a yam is a different starchy root vegetable. Yams are drier, have a starchier flesh, and dark, bark-like skin.

1 Pour 1 cup water into the inner pot of the Instant Pot® and place a steam rack inside. Place the sweet potato into a steamer basket and place it on top of the steam rack. Secure the lid.

2 Press the Manual or Pressure Cook button and adjust the time to 8 minutes.

3 When the timer beeps, quick-release pressure until float valve drops and then unlock lid.

4 Carefully remove the steamer basket from the inner pot and transfer the sweet potatoes to a large bowl.

5 Add the olive oil, thyme, rosemary, and garlic salt and use a potato masher to mash the potatoes to your desired consistency. Serve.

CALORIES: 110 | **FAT**: 4g | **PROTEIN**: 1g | **SODIUM**: 126mg
FIBER: 3g | **CARBOHYDRATES**: 17g | **SUGAR**: 3g

Mashed Cauliflower

Potato who? Cauliflower cooks and blends into a creamy, luscious stand-in for traditional mashed potatoes. Don't expect this dish to taste like potatoes—it doesn't. But rest assured it can stand on its own two legs and will likely become your new favorite side dish. In addition to the anti-inflammatory properties of cauliflower, the extra-virgin olive oil in this recipe will also provide protection against chronic inflammation. Virgin olive oil contains the phenolic compound oleocanthal, which has similar anti-inflammatory properties as ibuprofen.

- **Hands-On Time: 10 minutes**
- **Cook Time: 3 minutes**

Serves 4

1 large cauliflower crown, core removed and roughly chopped
2 cups chicken stock
2 tablespoons extra virgin olive oil plus ½ teaspoon for serving
½ teaspoon salt
½ teaspoon garlic powder
¾ cup nutritional yeast
¼ teaspoon freshly ground black pepper

WHY CHICKEN STOCK?

It may seem pointless to use chicken stock in this recipe when it isn't consumed at the end. It actually does serve a purpose, however, in that it adds tremendous flavor to the cauliflower when it's cooking in the Instant Pot®. Water just doesn't yield the same result!

1 Add the cauliflower and stock to the inner pot. Secure the lid.

2 Press the Manual or Pressure Cook button and adjust the time to 3 minutes.

3 When the timer beeps, quick-release pressure until float valve drops and then unlock lid.

4 Use a slotted spoon to transfer the cauliflower to a food processor. Add the 2 tablespoons oil, salt, garlic powder, and nutritional yeast to the food processor and process until silky smooth.

5 Transfer to a medium bowl, drizzle with ½ teaspoon olive oil, sprinkle with the pepper, and serve immediately.

CALORIES: 173 | FAT: 8g | PROTEIN: 11g | SODIUM: 414mg
FIBER: 7g | CARBOHYDRATES: 16g | SUGAR: 5g

7

Poultry Main Dishes

Everyone knows how important healthy dinners are. But getting a healthy dinner on the table is not always easy in today's world. Your dinners are about to become quicker and easier without sacrificing any flavor! The Instant Pot® can transform how you prepare your dinners, with less effort and more time to spend with your family.

If you think you have to eat a totally plant-based diet to fight inflammation, that's not true. Poultry can be a healthy part of an anti-inflammatory diet. Vegetables are still the most important part of any diet, but as long as you are including ample vegetables and other plant foods in your diet, you can consume poultry and still eat in a way that promotes a healthy inflammatory response in your body.

From one-pot wonders like Chicken, Mushrooms, and Quinoa to lifesavers like cooking a whole chicken in your Instant Pot® (see Whole "Roasted" Chicken in this chapter), you are going to be amazed at the flavor and time-saving dinners the recipes here provide you.

Asian Noodle Bowls

If you're craving noodles on an anti-inflammatory diet, brown rice noodles are the way to go. Brown rice noodles are gluten-free and will help maintain a balanced blood sugar level more than traditional white pasta. This recipe yields a sticky noodle and the starches thicken the sauce naturally.

- **Hands-On Time: 10 minutes**
- **Cook Time: 3 minutes**

Serves 4

½ cup reduced sodium tamari

2 tablespoons rice vinegar

2 tablespoons almond butter

2 tablespoons erythritol

2 cups chicken broth

1 pound boneless, skinless chicken breast, cut into bite-sized pieces

2 large carrots, peeled and thickly sliced (½") on the diagonal

8 ounces uncooked brown rice noodles

¼ cup sliced scallions

4 tablespoons chopped almonds

1 Place the tamari, vinegar, almond butter, erythritol, broth, chicken pieces, and carrots in the inner pot and then top with noodles. Secure the lid.

2 Press the Manual or Pressure Cook button and adjust the time to 3 minutes.

3 When the timer beeps, quick-release pressure until float valve drops and then unlock lid.

4 Carefully stir the ingredients. Portion into four bowls and top with scallions and a sprinkle of almonds.

CALORIES: 482 | **FAT**: 11g | **PROTEIN**: 36g | **SODIUM**: 1,392mg
FIBER: 5g | **CARBOHYDRATES**: 62g | **SUGAR**: 6g

Lemon Garlic Chicken Thighs

This simple recipe delivers on flavor in a big way, and boneless, skinless chicken thighs cook to tender perfection in the Instant Pot®. Resist the temptation to quick-release pressure after the cooking time. The key to perfectly cooked chicken in your Instant Pot®, that isn't dry in the least, is to let pressure release naturally. So be patient and the reward will be worth it!

- **Hands-On Time: 10 minutes**
- **Cook Time: 11 minutes**

Serves 4

1 tablespoon avocado oil
1½ pounds boneless, skinless chicken thighs
1 small onion, peeled and diced
1 tablespoon minced garlic
Juice and zest from 1 large lemon
1 tablespoon Italian seasoning blend
⅓ cup chicken stock
1 tablespoon arrowroot powder

1 Add the oil to the inner pot. Press the Sauté button and heat oil 2 minutes.

2 Place the chicken thighs in the inner pot and brown 2 minutes per side. Remove the chicken thighs from the pot and set aside.

3 Add the onion to the pot and sauté 2 minutes. Add the garlic and sauté another 30 seconds.

4 Add the lemon juice, lemon zest, and Italian seasoning. Scrape up any brown bits from the bottom of the pot. Press the Cancel button.

5 Put the chicken thighs back in the pot along with stock. Secure the lid.

6 Press the Manual or Pressure Cook button and adjust the time to 7 minutes.

7 When the timer beeps, let pressure release naturally until float valve drops and then unlock lid.

8 Remove the chicken from the pot and then stir in the arrowroot powder. When the sauce is thickened, serve on top of the chicken thighs.

CALORIES: 262 | **FAT**: 10g | **PROTEIN**: 34g | **SODIUM**: 190mg
FIBER: 1g | **CARBOHYDRATES**: 6g | **SUGAR**: 1g

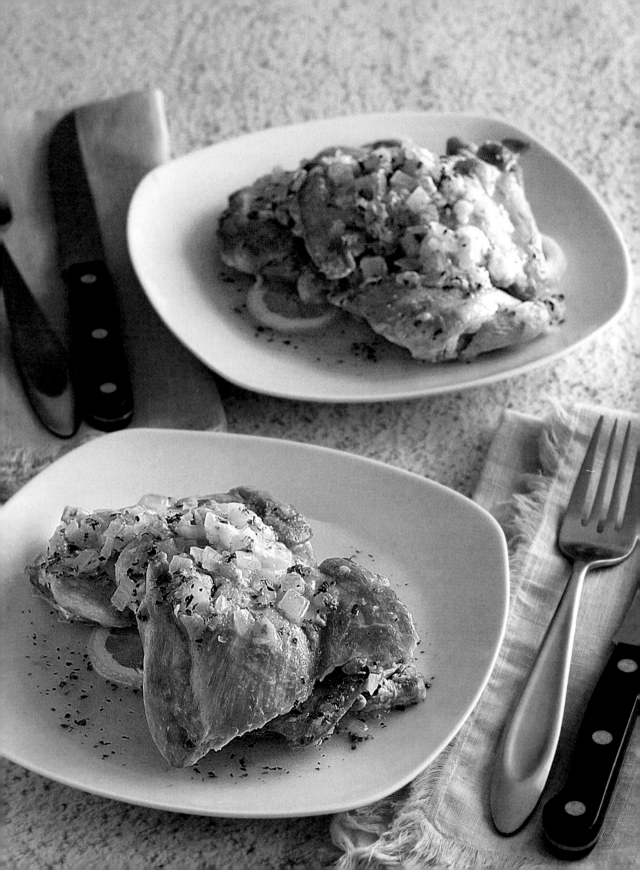

Creamy Coconut Lime Chicken Bowl with Cauliflower and Spinach

The rich flavor and creamy texture of this one-pot dinner will blow your mind. Full-fat coconut milk lends its best features to this dish, and lime, ginger, and cumin add to its outstanding flavor. There are a number of anti-inflammatory ingredients working together in this recipe, including the onion, cauliflower, coconut, ginger, and lime! You'll love the ease of having a one-pot dinner that is a hit with everyone.

- **Hands-On Time: 15 minutes**
- **Cook Time: 11 minutes**

Serves 4

1 tablespoon coconut oil

1 small yellow onion, peeled and diced

2 heaping cups large cauliflower florets

1½ pounds boneless, skinless chicken breasts, cut into 1½" chunks

1 (13.66-ounce) can unsweetened full-fat coconut milk

1 cup chicken broth

Juice from 1 medium lime

1 teaspoon kosher salt

1 teaspoon ground cumin

½ teaspoon ground ginger

2 cups baby spinach leaves

1　Press the Sauté button and add the oil to the inner pot. When the oil melts, add the onion and cook until it's softened, about 5 minutes.

2　Add the cauliflower, chicken, coconut milk, broth, lime juice, salt, cumin, and ginger and stir well to combine. Secure the lid.

3　Press the Manual or Pressure Cook button and adjust the time to 6 minutes.

4　When the timer beeps, let pressure release naturally until float valve drops and then unlock lid.

5　Stir in the spinach until it is wilted and then serve.

CALORIES: 457 | **FAT**: 26g | **PROTEIN**: 43g | **SODIUM**: 931mg
FIBER: 2g | **CARBOHYDRATES**: 9g | **SUGAR**: 2g

SIZE MATTERS

Make sure you don't cut your cauliflower florets too small or they will become mushy with the cooking time. Large florets will hold up well in this recipe.

Chicken, Mushroom, and Cauliflower Bake

Sometimes, you just need a dump-and-go dinner like this one. You place the ingredients in the Instant Pot® and let the machine work its magic. In a little while, you'll have a hot cooked meal ready to enjoy. Research shows that even small amounts of shiitake mushrooms can decrease inflammatory markers in the blood, so this dinner can have impressive anti-inflammatory benefits too.

- **Hands-On Time: 5 minutes**
- **Cook Time: 5 minutes**

Serves 4

4 cups riced cauliflower

8 ounces white mushrooms, chopped

8 ounces shiitake mushrooms, stems removed and chopped

8 ounces oyster mushrooms, chopped

1½ pounds boneless, skinless chicken breasts, cut into bite-sized pieces

¼ cup chicken stock

1 tablespoon minced garlic

1 teaspoon salt

1 teaspoon dried thyme

Juice from 1 large lemon

1 Place the cauliflower, mushrooms, and chicken in the inner pot of the Instant Pot®.

2 In a small bowl, whisk together the stock, garlic, salt, thyme, and lemon juice.

3 Pour the liquid over the ingredients in the Instant Pot® and stir to combine. Secure the lid.

4 Press the Manual or Pressure Cook button and adjust the time to 5 minutes.

5 When the timer beeps, let pressure release naturally until float valve drops and then unlock lid. Stir and serve.

CALORIES: 432 | **FAT**: 4g | **PROTEIN**: 50g | **SODIUM**: 428mg
FIBER: 11g | **CARBOHYDRATES**: 54g | **SUGAR**: 5g

Strawberry Avocado Salad with Chicken

Strawberries, avocados, chicken, and almond slices come together in a salad that is full of beautiful flavors and textures. What really makes this unique salad shine is the bright and vibrant strawberry vinaigrette that dresses it. Its pink color is stunning and this is sure to be the prettiest salad you ever make! More than beautiful, this salad also delivers an abundance of anti-inflammatory benefits. From the strawberries to the almonds, you are getting powerful nutrients in this delicious dinner.

- **Hands-On Time: 10 minutes**
- **Cook Time: 6 minutes**

Serves 4

1 pound boneless, skinless chicken breasts

½ cup chicken stock

13 large strawberries, hulled, divided

2 tablespoons extra-virgin olive oil

2 tablespoons fresh lemon juice

¼ teaspoon ground ginger

⅛ teaspoon white pepper

8 cups baby spinach

1 medium avocado, peeled, pitted, and cut into slices

⅓ cup sliced almonds

½ teaspoon salt

¼ teaspoon freshly ground black pepper

1 Add the chicken breasts and stock to the inner pot of the Instant Pot®. Secure the lid.

2 Press the Manual or Pressure Cook button and adjust the time to 6 minutes.

3 Meanwhile, make the dressing. In a blender, place five hulled strawberries, oil, lemon juice, ginger, and white pepper and blend until smooth. Set aside.

4 Slice the remaining eight strawberries, set aside.

5 When the timer beeps, let pressure release naturally until float valve drops and then unlock lid.

6 Remove the chicken from the Instant Pot® and allow it to cool completely. Once it is cool, chop the chicken.

7 In a large serving bowl, place the baby spinach, avocado slices, almonds, and strawberry slices. Add the chopped chicken. Drizzle with the salad dressing, add salt and pepper, and toss to combine.

CALORIES: 333 | **FAT**: 18g | **PROTEIN**: 33g | **SODIUM**: 392mg
FIBER: 6g | **CARBOHYDRATES**: 12g | **SUGAR**: 4g

Chicken, Mushrooms, and Quinoa

Chicken, mushrooms, and quinoa cook together for a hearty, casserole-like dish.

- **Hands-On Time: 15 minutes**
- **Cook Time: 5 minutes**

Serves 6

1 tablespoon avocado oil

1 small yellow onion, diced

6 cloves garlic, minced

1½ pounds boneless, skinless chicken thighs, cut into bite-sized pieces

2 (8-ounce) packages sliced white mushrooms

3 cups chicken stock

1½ cups quinoa, rinsed well

1 cup nondairy Greek-style yogurt

1 Add the oil to the inner pot. Press the Sauté button and heat the oil 1 minute. Add the onion and sauté 5 minutes. Add the garlic and sauté an additional 30 seconds. Press the Cancel button.

2 Add the chicken, mushrooms, stock, quinoa, and yogurt and stir to combine. Secure the lid.

3 Press the Manual or Pressure Cook button and adjust the time to 3 minutes.

4 When the timer beeps, quick-release pressure until float valve drops and then unlock lid.

5 Spoon onto plates or into bowls to serve.

CALORIES: 397 | FAT: 10g | PROTEIN: 37g | SODIUM: 294mg
FIBER: 4g | CARBOHYDRATES: 37g | SUGAR: 5g

Turkey Sweet Potato Hash

This versatile recipe can be breakfast or a make-ahead lunch option for work.

- **Hands-On Time: 10 minutes**
- **Cook Time: 17 minutes**

Serves 4

1½ tablespoons avocado oil

1 medium yellow onion, peeled and diced

2 cloves garlic, minced

1 medium sweet potato, cut into cubes (peeling not necessary)

½ pound lean ground turkey

½ teaspoon salt

1 teaspoon Italian seasoning blend

1 Press the Sauté button and add the oil. Allow the oil to heat 1 minute and then add the onion and cook until softened, about 5 minutes. Add the garlic and cook an additional 30 seconds.

2 Add the sweet potato, turkey, salt, and Italian seasoning and cook another 5 minutes. Press the Cancel button. Secure the lid.

3 Press the Manual or Pressure Cook button and adjust the time to 5 minutes.

4 When the timer beeps, quick-release pressure until float valve drops and then unlock lid. Spoon onto plates and serve.

CALORIES: 172 | FAT: 9g | PROTEIN: 12g | SODIUM: 348mg
FIBER: 1g | CARBOHYDRATES: 10g | SUGAR: 3g

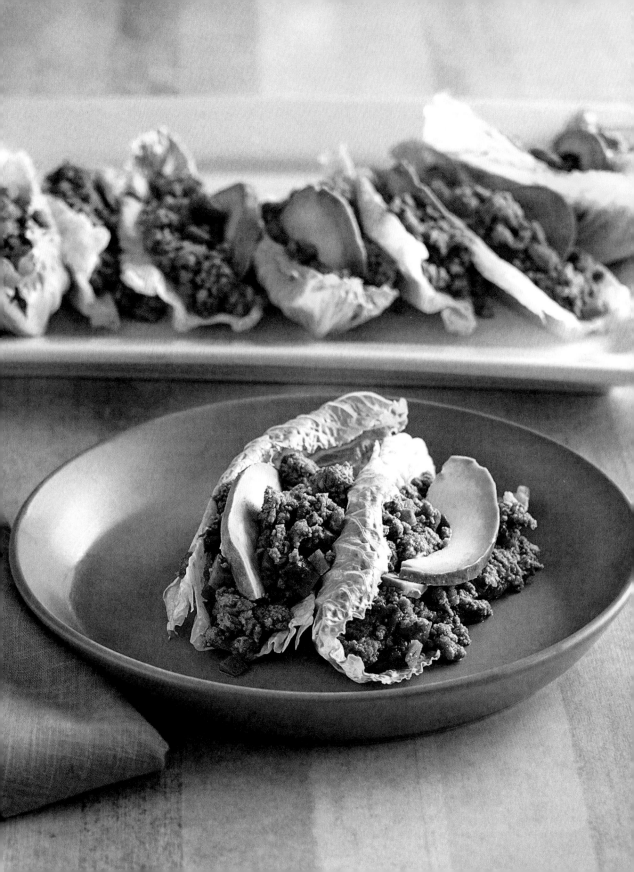

Turkey Taco Lettuce Boats

You'll never think about tacos the same way again after you've tried this recipe. Instead of taco shells, a large romaine lettuce leaf becomes home for all of your taco fixings. This is not only a healthy way to enjoy tacos, but the cool, crisp leaf is a nice contrast to the warm taco mixture.

- **Hands-On Time: 10 minutes**
- **Cook Time: 24 minutes**

Serves 4

1 tablespoon avocado oil

1 medium onion, peeled and diced

2 large carrots, peeled and diced

2 medium stalks celery, ends removed and diced

2 cloves garlic, minced

1 pound lean ground turkey

1 teaspoon chili powder

1 teaspoon paprika

1 teaspoon cumin

½ teaspoon salt

¼ teaspoon black pepper

1 cup chipotle salsa

12 large romaine leaves

1 medium avocado, peeled, pitted, and sliced

1 Press the Sauté button and add the oil. Allow the oil to heat 1 minute and then add the onion, carrots, celery, and garlic. Cook until softened, about 5 minutes.

2 Add the turkey and cook until browned, about 3 minutes.

3 Add the chili powder, paprika, cumin, salt, pepper, and salsa and stir to combine. Press the Cancel button. Secure the lid.

4 Press the Manual or Pressure Cook button and adjust the time to 15 minutes.

5 When the timer beeps, quick-release pressure until float valve drops and then unlock lid.

6 To serve, spoon a portion of the taco meat into a romaine lettuce leaf and then top with sliced avocado.

CALORIES: 339 | FAT: 18g | PROTEIN: 27g | SODIUM: 900mg
FIBER: 8g | CARBOHYDRATES: 18g | SUGAR: 8g

Turkey and Greens Meatloaf

No more worrying that you won't have time for the meatloaf to cook on a busy weeknight—the Instant Pot® shaves a good portion of the normal cooking time off! Adding greens to your turkey meatloaf is a brilliant way to get more nutrient-dense greens into your diet. Your picky eaters might not even mind with this moist and flavorful meatloaf!

- **Hands-On Time: 15 minutes**
- **Cook Time: 25 minutes**

Serves 4

1 tablespoon avocado oil

1 small onion, peeled and diced

2 cloves garlic, minced

3 cups mixed baby greens, finely chopped

1 pound lean ground turkey

¼ cup almond flour

1 large egg

¾ teaspoon salt

½ teaspoon black pepper

1 Add the oil to the inner pot. Press the Sauté button and heat the oil 1 minute.

2 Add the onion and sauté until softened, 3 minutes. Add the garlic and greens and sauté 1 more minute. Press the Cancel button.

3 In a medium bowl, combine the turkey, flour, egg, salt, and pepper.

4 Add the onion and greens mixture to the turkey mixture and stir to combine.

5 Rinse out the inner pot and then add 2 cups water.

6 Make an aluminum foil sling by folding a large piece of foil in half and bending the edges upward.

7 Form the turkey mixture into a rectangular loaf and place it on the aluminum foil sling. Place the sling onto the steam rack with handles, and lower it into the inner pot. Secure the lid.

8 Press the Manual or Pressure Cook button and adjust the time to 20 minutes.

9 When the timer beeps, quick-release pressure until float valve drops and then unlock lid.

10 Carefully remove the meatloaf from the inner pot and allow it to rest for 10 minutes before slicing to serve.

CALORIES: 271 | FAT: 17g | PROTEIN: 25g | SODIUM: 406mg
FIBER: 2g | CARBOHYDRATES: 5g | SUGAR: 1g

Simple Italian Seasoned Turkey Breast

Don't save the turkey for Thanksgiving. This simple recipe will have you craving a Thanksgiving turkey all year long. The Instant Pot® produces a perfectly moist and tender turkey breast in a fraction of the time it takes to cook in the oven!

- **Hands-On Time: 10 minutes**
- **Cook Time: 18 minutes**

Serves 4

1½ pounds boneless, skinless turkey breast

2 tablespoons avocado oil, divided

1 teaspoon sweet paprika

1 teaspoon Italian seasoning blend

½ teaspoon kosher salt

½ teaspoon thyme

¼ teaspoon garlic salt

¼ teaspoon black pepper

1 Dry the turkey breast with a towel. Cut the turkey breast in half to fit in your Instant Pot®.

2 Brush both sides of the turkey breast with 1 tablespoon oil.

3 In a small bowl, mix together the paprika, Italian seasoning, kosher salt, thyme, garlic salt, and pepper. Rub this mixture onto both sides of the turkey breast.

4 Press the Sauté button and heat the remaining 1 tablespoon oil in the inner pot 2 minutes. Add the turkey breast and sear it on both sides, about 3 minutes per side. Press the Cancel button.

5 Remove the turkey from the inner pot and place it on a plate. Add 1 cup water to the inner pot and use a spatula to scrape up any brown bits that are stuck. Place the steam rack in the pot and the turkey breast on top of it. Secure the lid.

6 Press the Manual or Pressure Cook button and adjust the time to 10 minutes.

7 When the timer beeps, let pressure release naturally until float valve drops and then unlock lid. Slice and serve.

CALORIES: 248 | **FAT**: 9g | **PROTEIN**: 40g | **SODIUM**: 568mg
FIBER: 0g | **CARBOHYDRATES**: 0g | **SUGAR**: 0g

Spiced Chicken and Vegetables

This chicken dishes utilizes a bold seasoning blend to make a flavorful dinner that is quick and easy to prepare. This dish is wonderful served with Basic Brown Rice or Coconut Curry Lentils (see recipes in Chapter 5).

- **Hands-On Time: 15 minutes**
- **Cook Time: 15 minutes**

Serves 4

1 teaspoon dried thyme
¼ teaspoon ground ginger
¼ teaspoon ground allspice
1 teaspoon kosher salt
½ teaspoon black pepper
2 large bone-in chicken breasts (about 2 pounds)
½ cup chicken stock
2 medium onions, peeled and cut in fourths
4 medium carrots

1   In a small bowl, mix together the thyme, ginger, allspice, salt, and pepper.

2   Use half of the spice mixture to season the chicken breasts.

3   Pour the chicken stock into the inner pot and then add the chicken breasts. Place the onions and carrots on top of the chicken and sprinkle them with the rest of the seasoning blend. Secure the lid.

4   Press the Manual or Pressure Cook button and adjust the time to 15 minutes.

5   When the timer beeps, let pressure release naturally until float valve drops and then unlock lid.

6   Remove the chicken and the vegetables and serve alone or with rice or lentils.

CALORIES: 337 | FAT: 5g | PROTEIN: 56g | SODIUM: 755mg
FIBER: 3g | CARBOHYDRATES: 12g | SUGAR: 5g

Lemon Garlic Turkey Breast

Turkey breasts are so quick and easy to make in the Instant Pot®, it's worth trying a variety of different flavor combinations. This recipe uses lemon and garlic, a classic combination. Lemon zest brightens the flavor, and garlic and shallot add complexity. The whole family will love the taste of this dinner, and you'll love the ease of preparing it.

- **Hands-On Time: 10 minutes**
- **Cook Time: 17 minutes**

Serves 4

1 (1½-pound) boneless, skinless turkey breast

2 tablespoons avocado oil, divided

Zest from ½ large lemon

½ medium shallot, peeled and minced

1 large clove garlic, minced

½ teaspoon kosher salt

¼ teaspoon black pepper

1 Dry the turkey breast with a towel. Cut the turkey breast in half to fit in your Instant Pot®.

2 Brush both sides of the turkey breast with 1 tablespoon oil.

3 In a small bowl, mix together the lemon zest, shallot, garlic, salt, and pepper. Rub this mixture onto both sides of the turkey breast.

4 Press the Sauté button and heat the remaining 1 tablespoon oil in the inner pot 2 minutes. Add the turkey breast and sear it on both sides, about 3 minutes per side. Press the Cancel button.

5 Remove the turkey from the inner pot and place it on a plate. Add 1 cup water to the inner pot and use a spatula to scrape up any brown bits that are stuck. Place the steam rack in the pot and the turkey breast on top of it. Secure the lid.

6 Press the Manual or Pressure Cook button and adjust the time to 10 minutes.

7 When the timer beeps, let pressure release naturally until float valve drops and then unlock lid. Slice and serve.

CALORIES: 250 | FAT: 9g | PROTEIN: 40g | SODIUM: 445mg
FIBER: 0g | CARBOHYDRATES: 1g | SUGAR: 0g

Homestyle Chicken and Vegetables

Homestyle Chicken and Vegetables is always a family-favorite dinner. Now you can make it so much quicker by using your Instant Pot® pressure cooker. The bone-in chicken breasts stay moist and tender and the carrots and potatoes cook at the same time in the same pot. Those bright orange carrots also have vitamin A and beta-carotene, both of which are believed to be potent inflammation fighters. Dinnertime has never been easier or more delicious.

- **Hands-On Time: 5 minutes**
- **Cook Time: 15 minutes**

Serves 4

2 large bone-in chicken breasts (about 2 pounds)

1 teaspoon kosher salt, divided

½ teaspoon black pepper, divided

½ cup chicken stock

6 large carrots

8 medium whole new potatoes

1 Season the chicken breasts with $1/2$ teaspoon salt and $1/4$ teaspoon pepper.

2 Pour the stock into the inner pot and then add the chicken breasts. Place the carrots and potatoes on top of the chicken and season them with the rest of the salt and pepper. Secure the lid.

3 Press the Manual or Pressure Cook button and adjust the time to 15 minutes.

4 When the timer beeps, let pressure release naturally until float valve drops and then unlock lid.

5 Transfer to plates to serve and spoon the juices on top.

CALORIES: 398 | **FAT:** 5g | **PROTEIN:** 58g | **SODIUM:** 822mg
FIBER: 5g | **CARBOHYDRATES:** 24g | **SUGAR:** 6g

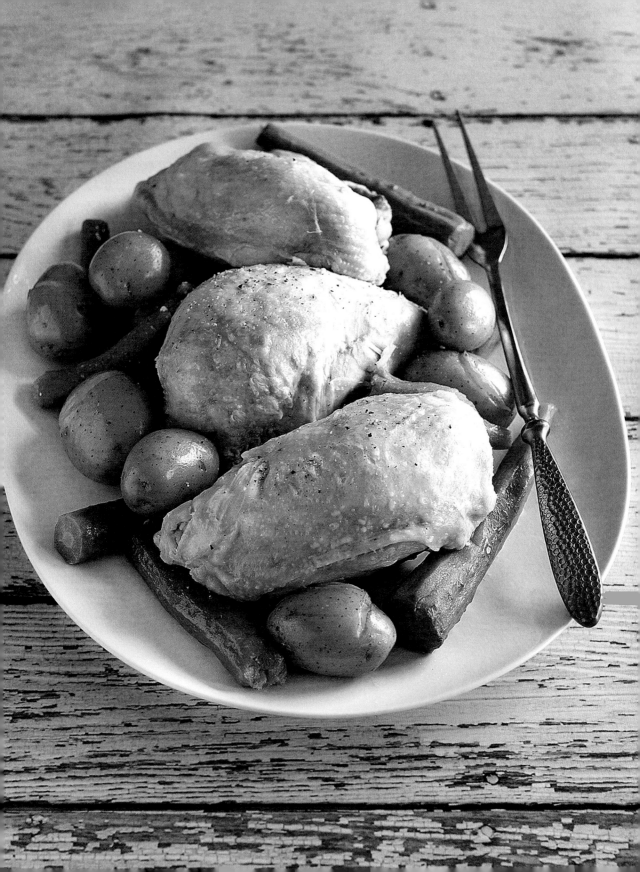

Chicken Tenders with Honey Mustard Sauce

Everything is better with a tasty dipping sauce, and this recipe is no exception. These chicken tenders cook quickly and perfectly in the Instant Pot® and they are made even better with a simple two-ingredient dipping sauce. This is a kid-friendly dinner that the whole family will enjoy.

- **Hands-On Time: 5 minutes**
- **Cook Time: 7 minutes**

Serves 4

1 pound chicken tenders
1 tablespoon fresh thyme leaves
½ teaspoon salt
¼ teaspoon black pepper
1 tablespoon avocado oil
1 cup chicken stock
¼ cup Dijon mustard
¼ cup raw honey

THE HEALTH BENEFITS OF RAW HONEY

Raw honey is rich in antioxidants so seek it out over processed honey where many of the nutrients have been destroyed. If your raw honey is thick or grainy, use an immersion blender to make the sauce more smooth.

1 Dry the chicken tenders with a towel and then season them with the thyme, salt, and pepper.

2 Press the Sauté button and then use the Adjust button to change to the More setting. Add the oil to the inner pot and let it heat 2 minutes. Add the chicken tenders and seer them until brown on both sides, about 1 minute per side. Press the Cancel button.

3 Remove the chicken tenders and set aside. Add the stock to the pot. Use a spoon to scrape up any small bits from the bottom of the pot.

4 Place the steam rack in the inner pot and place the chicken tenders directly on the rack. Secure the lid.

5 Press the Manual or Pressure Cook button and adjust the time to 3 minutes.

6 While the chicken is cooking, make the honey mustard sauce. In a small bowl, combine the Dijon mustard and honey and stir to combine.

7 When the timer beeps, let pressure release naturally until float valve drops and then unlock lid. Serve the chicken tenders with the honey mustard sauce.

CALORIES: 223 | **FAT**: 5g | **PROTEIN**: 22g | **SODIUM**: 778mg
FIBER: 0g | **CARBOHYDRATES**: 19g | **SUGAR**: 18g

Chicken Breasts with Cabbage and Mushrooms

If you think boneless, skinless chicken breasts have to be bland or boring, think again. Cabbage and mushrooms provide a savory punch to this one-pot meal. Cabbage and mushrooms also both have inflammation-fighting compounds, making this meal perfect for your anti-inflammatory diet.

- **Hands-On Time: 10 minutes**
- **Cook Time: 18 minutes**

Serves 4

2 tablespoons avocado oil
1 pound sliced baby bella mushrooms
1½ teaspoons salt, divided
2 cloves garlic, minced
8 cups chopped green cabbage
1½ teaspoons dried thyme
½ cup chicken stock
1½ pounds boneless, skinless chicken breasts

1 Press the Sauté button. Add the oil to the inner pot and allow it to heat 1 minute. Add the mushrooms and ¼ teaspoon salt and sauté until they have cooked down and released their liquid, about 10 minutes.

2 Add the garlic and sauté another 30 seconds. Press the Cancel button.

3 Add the cabbage, ¼ teaspoon salt, thyme, and stock to the inner pot and stir to combine.

4 Dry the chicken breasts and sprinkle both sides with the remaining salt. Place on top of the cabbage mixture. Secure the lid.

5 Press the Manual or Pressure Cook button and adjust the time to 6 minutes.

6 When the timer beeps, let pressure release naturally for 10 minutes, then quick-release any remaining pressure until float valve drops, then unlock lid.

7 Transfer to plates and spoon the juices on top.

CALORIES: 337 | **FAT**: 10g | **PROTEIN**: 44g | **SODIUM**: 1,023mg
FIBER: 4g | **CARBOHYDRATES**: 14g | **SUGAR**: 2g

Coconut Lime Chicken and Rice

Chicken and rice is a classic favorite, and here it's given a little bit of Caribbean flair. Coconut milk gives this dish a creamy, rich texture. While full-fat coconut milk adds the most flavor, the lite version works as well. Dried ginger adds spice to this recipe, but that's not all. Ginger contains gingerols, which posses powerful anti-inflammatory and antioxidant properties.

- **Hands-On Time: 5 minutes**
- **Cook Time: 5 minutes**

Serves 4

1 cup jasmine rice

1 (13.66-ounce) can unsweetened full-fat coconut milk

½ cup chicken stock

1¼ pounds boneless, skinless chicken breasts, cut into 1" cubes

1 teaspoon salt

½ teaspoon ground cumin

¼ teaspoon ground ginger

Juice from 1 medium lime

½ cup chopped cilantro leaves and stems

1 Place the rice, coconut milk, stock, chicken, salt, cumin, and ginger in the inner pot and stir to combine. Secure the lid.

2 Press the Manual or Pressure Cook button and adjust the time to 5 minutes.

3 When the timer beeps, let pressure release naturally for 10 minutes, then quick-release any remaining pressure until float valve drops, then unlock lid.

4 Stir in the lime juice and spoon into four bowls. Top each bowl with an equal amount of cilantro and serve.

CALORIES: 527 | **FAT**: 22g | **PROTEIN**: 38g | **SODIUM**: 702mg
FIBER: 1g | **CARBOHYDRATES**: 38g | **SUGAR**: 1g

Whole "Roasted" Chicken

The amazing Instant Pot® is able to cook a whole chicken in less than 30 minutes. Your meal-prep Sunday just got a whole lot easier. Use the cooked chicken in this recipe to supplement your dinners or lunches for the week. You can shred it or chop it and it can be added to salads, soups, or any recipe that calls for cooked chicken. Don't forget to make your homemade bone broth when you're finished!

- **Hands-On Time: 5 minutes**
- **Cook Time: 28 minutes**

Serves 6

¾ cup water
1 medium lemon
1 (4-pound) whole chicken
1 tablespoon salt
2 teaspoons black pepper

HOW TO ACCOUNT FOR DIFFERENT-SIZED BIRDS

If you happen to buy a whole chicken that is a little smaller or larger than the 4 pound chicken that the recipe calls for, simply adjust the time according to this formula: Cook a whole chicken for 7 minutes per pound.

1 Add water to the inner pot.

2 Cut the lemon in half. Squeeze the juice of half the lemon onto the chicken and sprinkle with salt and pepper. Stuff the other half of the lemon inside the bird.

3 Place the chicken in the pot breast side down. Secure the lid.

4 Press the Manual or Pressure Cook button and adjust the time to 28 minutes.

5 When the timer beeps, let pressure release naturally until float valve drops and then unlock lid.

6 Carefully remove the chicken from the inner pot and allow it to rest 10 minutes before slicing to serve.

CALORIES: 341 | **FAT**: 20g | **PROTEIN**: 32g | **SODIUM**: 1,249mg
FIBER: 0g | **CARBOHYDRATES**: 1g | **SUGAR**: 0g

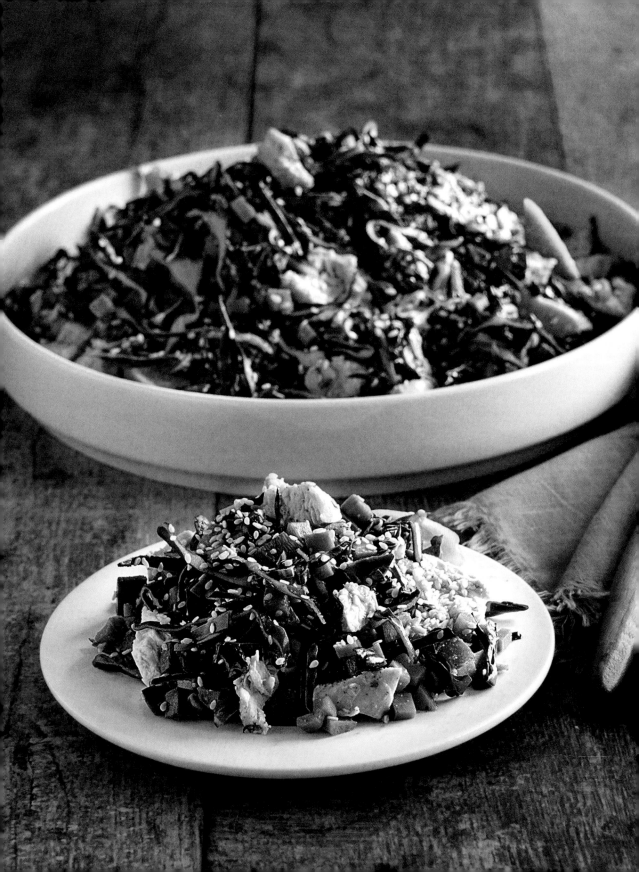

Asian Chopped Kale Salad with Chicken

A 1-cup serving of kale gives you over 1,000 percent of the amount of vitamin K you need in a day. Vitamin K is important for bone health and heart health, and it also helps maintain brain function and a healthy metabolism. They don't call kale a superfood without good reason. When it's chopped finely and dressed with this addicting Asian dressing, you will forget you're eating something so nutritious!

- **Hands-On Time: 20 minutes**
- **Cook Time: 6 minutes**

Serves 4

1 pound boneless, skinless chicken breast

½ cup chicken stock

2 bunches kale (about 12 ounces total), deveined and finely chopped

1 medium red bell pepper, seeded and diced

1 cup diced carrot

3 cups chopped cabbage

¼ cup pure sesame oil

¼ cup almond butter

¼ cup raw honey

Juice from 2 medium limes

1 tablespoon reduced sodium tamari

¼ teaspoon minced garlic

⅓ cup sesame seeds

1 Add the chicken breasts and stock to the inner pot of the Instant Pot®. Secure the lid.

2 Press the Manual or Pressure Cook button and adjust the time to 6 minutes.

3 When the timer beeps, let pressure release naturally until float valve drops and then unlock lid.

4 Remove the chicken from the Instant Pot® and allow it to cool completely. Once it is cool, chop the chicken.

5 In a large bowl, mix together the kale, bell peppers, carrots, cabbage, and chopped chicken.

6 In a blender, blend together the oil, almond butter, honey, lime juice, tamari, and garlic until smooth. Pour the dressing onto the kale salad and toss to coat. Add the sesame seeds and lightly toss. Serve.

CALORIES: 561 | **FAT**: 30g | **PROTEIN**: 36g | **SODIUM**: 332mg
FIBER: 9g | **CARBOHYDRATES**: 41g | **SUGAR**: 25g

**PERFECT
MEAL-PREP LUNCH**

This recipe works very well for a meal-prep lunch. You can't go wrong when you can cook once and eat a delicious meal for the next three days!

Jerk Chicken

Transport yourself to Jamaica with this flavorful chicken recipe. For the most authentic and spicy flavor, don't totally deseed your peppers. Leave a few seeds to bring up the heat, the spicier you like it, the more seeds you should leave. This is wonderful with rice and a large green salad.

- **Hands-On Time: 15 minutes**
- **Cook Time: 22 minutes**

Serves 8

1 large onion, peeled and cut into 8 pieces
1 tablespoon peeled and chopped fresh ginger
3 small hot chili peppers, deveined and deseeded
½ teaspoon ground allspice
2 tablespoons dry mustard
1 teaspoon black pepper
2 tablespoons red wine vinegar
2 tablespoons coconut aminos
2 cloves garlic, minced
½ cup chicken stock
4 pounds boneless, skinless chicken breasts cut in 1" pieces

1 Combine all ingredients except the chicken in a food processor or blender and process until liquefied.

2 Add the chicken to the Instant Pot®, top with the sauce, and stir to combine. Secure the lid.

3 Press the Manual or Pressure Cook button and adjust the time to 12 minutes.

4 When the timer beeps, quick-release pressure until float valve drops and then unlock lid.

5 Remove the chicken from Instant Pot® and spread on a baking sheet lined with parchment paper or a silicone baking mat. Drizzle sauce over the chicken.

6 Serve as is, or for a golden-browned finish, set broiler to high and broil 6–10 minutes, turning once until chicken is nicely browned.

CALORIES: 306 | FAT: 5g | PROTEIN: 52g | SODIUM: 210mg
FIBER: 1g | CARBOHYDRATES: 6g | SUGAR: 2g

Avocado Chicken Salad

Regular chicken salad gets a major upgrade by using avocado in place of mayonnaise. The avocado adds tremendous creaminess, and celery gives that nice contrast of texture. Avocados are an excellent source of both heart-healthy monounsaturated fat and powerful antioxidants, which can help promote a positive inflammatory response in your body. Eat this recipe on a bed a fresh baby greens for an absolutely perfect lunch or light dinner.

- **Hands-On Time: 10 minutes**
- **Cook Time: 6 minutes**

Serves 4

1 pound boneless, skinless chicken breasts

½ cup chicken stock

1½ medium avocados, peeled, pitted, and mashed (1 cup mashed)

1 medium stalk celery, ends removed and diced

1 scallion, thinly sliced

1 tablespoon lemon juice

1 tablespoon chopped fresh parsley

½ teaspoon dried dill weed

2 teaspoons Dijon mustard

½ teaspoon kosher salt

¼ teaspoon freshly ground black pepper

1 Add the chicken breasts and stock to the inner pot of the Instant Pot®. Secure the lid.

2 Press the Manual or Pressure Cook button and adjust the time to 6 minutes.

3 When the timer beeps, let pressure release naturally until float valve drops and then unlock lid.

4 Remove the chicken from the Instant Pot® and allow it to cool completely. Once it is cool, chop the chicken.

5 Place the chopped chicken in a medium bowl and add the rest of the ingredients. Stir to combine.

CALORIES: 230 | FAT: 9g | PROTEIN: 27g | SODIUM: 421mg
FIBER: 4g | CARBOHYDRATES: 6g | SUGAR: 1g

Seafood and Fish Main Dishes

Fish and seafood are low-fat, high-protein, and provide you with a number of health benefits. White-fleshed fish is one of the lowest fat sources of animal protein you can consume. Oily fish, on the other hand, provides you with omega-3 fatty acids. These are some of the best fats you can consume and are considered anti-inflammatory.

Fish is also quite easy to prepare and quick to cook, making it an ideal choice for busy people who are committed to healthy eating. The Instant Pot® offers a number of advantages as the ideal cooking tool for all your fish and seafood meals. Not only are nutrients and flavors locked in using the pressure cooking method, but so are the smells. The worst part about cooking fish is having your entire house smell fishy while you're cooking it and for hours after. The Instant Pot® eliminates that problem!

Basic Shrimp

This is a great recipe to have in your back pocket whenever you need a quick protein to add to any dish. While your Instant Pot® is building pressure, you can quickly throw together a salad or vegetable side dish, and by the time your shrimp is cooked, dinner is ready. It doesn't get any easier than that.

- **Hands-On Time: 1 minute**
- **Cook Time: 0 minutes**

Serves 2

12 frozen jumbo shrimp, in shells

1 Pour 1½ cups water into the inner pot and place the steam rack inside. Add the shrimp to the steamer basket and place it on the rack. Secure the lid.

2 Press the Manual or Pressure Cook button and adjust the time to 0 minutes.

3 When the timer beeps, quick-release pressure until float valve drops and then unlock lid.

CALORIES: 80 | FAT: 1g | PROTEIN: 15g | SODIUM: 641mg
FIBER: 0g | CARBOHYDRATES: 1g | SUGAR: 0g

Garlic Shrimp and Broccoli

Garlic lovers will go crazy for this recipe! This recipe is loaded with garlic, but one of the best parts about using an Instant Pot® to cook is that your entire house won't smell like garlic when you are cooking this dish. Not only that, but you also won't smell fish or broccoli, two other ingredients that are notorious for smelling up houses.

- **Hands-On Time: 15 minutes**
- **Cook Time: 5 minutes**

Serves 4

2 tablespoons avocado oil
2 medium shallots, peeled and diced
1 tablespoon minced garlic
¾ cup chicken stock
1½ tablespoons lemon juice
½ teaspoon kosher salt
½ teaspoon black pepper
1½ pounds peeled, deveined jumbo shrimp
2½ cups small broccoli florets

TIME-SAVING TIP

Sometimes, convenience food isn't so bad! To reduce the prep time on this recipe, buy precut broccoli florets and shrimp that is already peeled and deveined.

1 Press the Sauté button and add the oil to the inner pot. Allow it to heat 1 minute and then add the shallots. Cook the shallots 3 minutes and then add the garlic and continue to cook an additional 1 minute.

2 Add the stock and use a spoon to remove any brown bits that are stuck to the pot.

3 Add the lemon juice, salt, pepper, and shrimp. Then add the broccoli to the top layer and do not stir. Secure the lid.

4 Press the Manual or Pressure Cook button and adjust the time to 0 minutes.

5 When the timer beeps, quick-release pressure until float valve drops and then unlock lid.

CALORIES: 231 | FAT: 9g | PROTEIN: 26g | SODIUM: 1,337mg
FIBER: 2g | CARBOHYDRATES: 10g | SUGAR: 3g

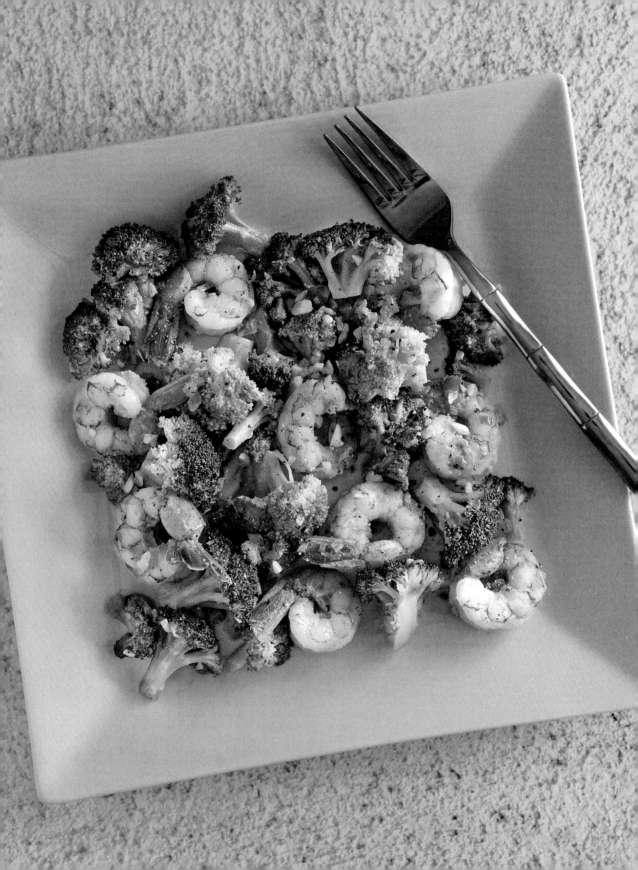

Shrimp Paella

If you always keep a bag of frozen shrimp in your freezer, this will be the perfect dinner for you on busy weeknights. This is a dinner that takes little prep besides adding your ingredients to the Instant Pot®—it doesn't get any better than that! Not only is it one of the easiest dinners to prepare, the turmeric in it is a power anti-inflammatory spice, making this dish a double win!

- **Hands-On Time: 7 minutes**
- **Cook Time: 14 minutes**

Serves 4

2 tablespoons avocado oil
1 medium white onion, peeled and chopped
4 cloves garlic, chopped
1 teaspoon paprika
1 teaspoon turmeric
½ teaspoon salt
¼ teaspoon black pepper
Pinch saffron threads
¼ teaspoon red pepper flakes
1 cup jasmine rice
1 cup chicken stock
1 pound frozen jumbo shrimp, shell and tail on
¼ cup chopped fresh cilantro

1 Press the Sauté button and add the oil to the inner pot. Allow it to heat 2 minutes, and then add the onion and cook until softened, about 5 minutes.

2 Add the garlic, paprika, turmeric, salt, black pepper, saffron, and red pepper flakes and sauté another 30 seconds. Add the rice, stir, and cook 1 more minute.

3 Add the stock and stir, and use a spoon to make sure there are no brown bits stuck to the bottom of the pot. Add the shrimp. Secure the lid.

4 Press the Manual or Pressure Cook button and adjust the time to 5 minutes.

5 When the timer beeps, quick-release pressure until float valve drops and then unlock lid.

6 Remove the mixture from the pot and peel the shrimp if desired.

7 Serve garnished with cilantro.

CALORIES: 331 | **FAT**: 9g | **PROTEIN**: 20g | **SODIUM**: 980mg
FIBER: 1g | **CARBOHYDRATES**: 41g | **SUGAR**: 2g

Strawberry Shrimp Salad

This recipe will prove to you that you can make restaurant-quality salads without leaving your house and for a fraction of the cost. Start with frozen, shell-on shrimp for the best texture, and a quick sauté at the end gives that lovely browning. Strawberries add a fresh, light component to this salad, but they are also an excellent source of vitamin C, which helps promote healthy inflammation in the body.

- **Hands-On Time: 15 minutes**
- **Cook Time: 0 minutes**

Serves 2

¼ cup extra-virgin olive oil

¼ cup apple cider vinegar

2 tablespoons fresh lemon juice

1 tablespoon raw honey

1 tablespoon Dijon mustard

1 clove garlic, minced

¼ teaspoon salt

¼ teaspoon black pepper

12 frozen jumbo shrimp

1 teaspoon Montreal steak seasoning

1 tablespoon avocado oil

8 cups mixed spring greens

⅔ cup chopped jicama

1½ cups sliced strawberries

⅔ cup pecans

1 In a small container or jar with a tight lid, add the olive oil, vinegar, lemon juice, honey, mustard, garlic, salt, and pepper and shake until the ingredients are well combined. Set aside.

2 Pour 1½ cups water into the inner pot and place the steam rack inside. Add the shrimp to the steamer basket and place it on the rack. Secure the lid.

3 Press the Manual or Pressure Cook button and adjust the time to 0 minutes.

4 When the timer beeps, quick-release pressure until float valve drops and then unlock lid. Carefully remove the steamer basket from the inner pot.

5 Peel the shrimp and place them in a medium bowl. Add the steak seasoning and gently toss to coat the shrimp in the seasoning.

6 Remove the water from the inner pot and wipe it dry. Press the Sauté button and use the Adjust button to change to the More setting.

7 Add the avocado oil to the inner pot and allow it to heat 1 minute. Add the shrimp and cook to brown, 1 minute per side.

8 Put the greens, jicama, strawberries, pecans, and shrimp in a large bowl. Drizzle with the dressing and toss gently to coat.

CALORIES: 742 | **FAT**: 57g | **PROTEIN**: 22g | **SODIUM**: 1,556mg
FIBER: 11g | **CARBOHYDRATES**: 34g | **SUGAR**: 18g

Lemon Dill Salmon

Salmon is one of the best sources of omega-3 fatty acids. These are essential fats that are beneficial for your heart health and brain health, and also help promote healthy inflammatory responses in your body. This recipe is a simple and classic flavoring for fish—lemon and dill. Serve with Lemony Steamed Asparagus (see recipe in Chapter 6) for a light and healthy meal.

- **Hands-On Time: 2 minutes**
- **Cook Time: 3 minutes**

Serves 4

4 (4", 6-ounce) salmon filets
1 teaspoon avocado oil
Juice of 1 medium lemon
1 teaspoon dried dill weed
½ teaspoon salt

WILD VERSUS FARMED SALMON

Even if you have to buy it frozen, it's worth seeking out wild-caught salmon. Farmed salmon is often fed a diet of genetically modified grains and injected with dyes to give the color it doesn't get from eating its natural diet.

1 Brush the salmon filets with oil, then top with the lemon juice, dill weed, and salt.

2 Add 1 cup water to the Instant Pot® and place the steam rack inside. Place the salmon filets on top of the steam rack. Secure the lid.

3 Press the Manual or Pressure Cook button and adjust the time to 3 minutes.

4 When the timer beeps, quick-release pressure until float valve drops and then unlock lid. Serve immediately.

CALORIES: 227 | **FAT**: 6g | **PROTEIN**: 35g | **SODIUM**: 418mg
FIBER: 0g | **CARBOHYDRATES**: 1g | **SUGAR**: 0g

Halibut in Parchment

Halibut is a rich source of selenium, which helps build your immune system, and helps fight against free radical damage and inflammation in your body. Halibut is nutritious and has a mild flavor and a quick cook time. Parchment paper locks in both moisture and flavor.

- **Hands-On Time: 5 minutes**
- **Cook Time: 3 minutes**

Serves 2

¼ teaspoon dried dill weed
1 tablespoon Dijon mustard
1 tablespoon chicken stock
1 teaspoon avocado oil
1 medium lemon
2 (5-ounce, 1"-thick) halibut filets

1 Cut two large pieces of parchment paper (about 15" by 16") and fold them in half width-wise. Set aside.

2 In a small bowl, whisk together the dill weed, mustard, stock, and oil.

3 Cut the lemon in half. Slice half of it and juice the other half; set the juice aside.

4 Unfold a piece of parchment paper and place one halibut filet on one side of the crease.

5 Pour 1 tablespoon lemon juice over the halibut and then top with half of the mustard-dill sauce and then add half of the lemon slices.

6 Fold the opposite side of the parchment paper over the side with the fish. Make small overlapping pleats to seal the open sides and create a half-moon-shaped packet. Make sure to press each crease as you fold. Repeat so you have two parchment packs.

7 Pour 1 cup water into the Instant Pot® and place the steam rack inside.

8 Place the parchment packets in a 7-cup round bowl and add aluminum foil to the top and place the bowl on top of the steam rack. Secure the lid.

9 Press the Manual or Pressure Cook button and adjust the time to 3 minutes.

10 When the timer beeps, quick-release pressure until float valve drops and then unlock lid. Serve the halibut in the parchment packets.

CALORIES: 167 | **FAT**: 4g | **PROTEIN**: 27g | **SODIUM**: 294mg
FIBER: 0g | **CARBOHYDRATES**: 1g | **SUGAR**: 0g

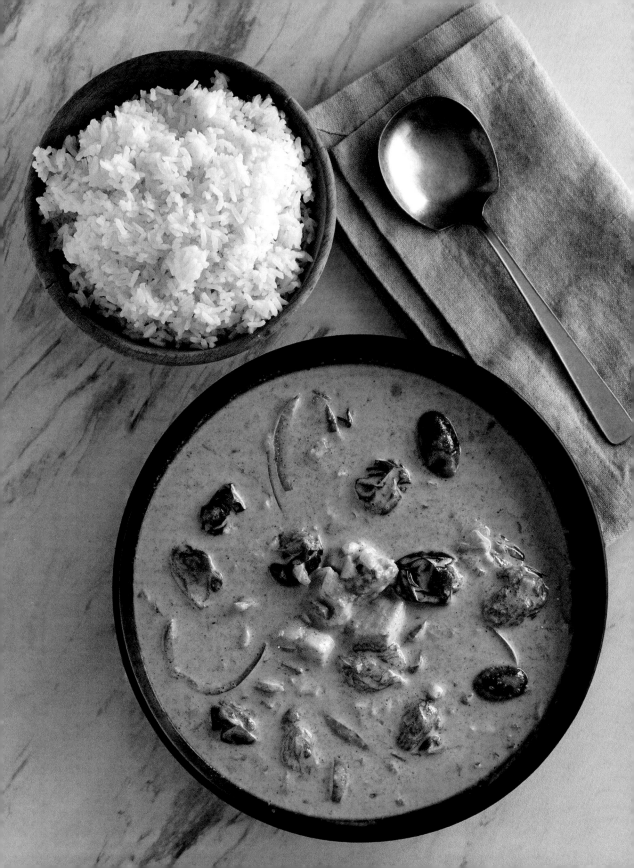

Coconut Fish Curry

Get ready for a flavor explosion with this fish recipe. Even the most reluctant fish eaters are sure to love this spicy curry dish. This can be eaten as a fish stew or served on a bed of jasmine rice. If you are sensitive to nightshades, you can eliminate the tomatoes from this recipe and the final result will still be amazing.

- **Hands-On Time: 10 minutes**
- **Cook Time: 14 minutes**

Serves 4

2 tablespoons avocado oil
6 large Thai basil leaves
1 large white onion, peeled and diced
1½ teaspoons salt
2 cloves garlic, minced
1 tablespoon peeled and grated fresh ginger
3 tablespoons curry powder
2 cups canned unsweetened full-fat coconut milk
2 green chilies, seeded and sliced into strips
1 cup whole cherry tomatoes
1½ pounds tilapia filet, cut into small pieces
2 tablespoons lemon juice

THAI BASIL

Most people are aware of Italian basil, but not as familiar with Thai basil. Thai basil has purple stems and narrower leaves than Italian basil. You can't really substitute one for the other as they have different flavor profiles.

1 Press the Sauté button and add the oil to the inner pot. Allow it to heat 1 minute, and then add the basil leaves and cook until they turn golden around the edges, about 1 minute.

2 Add the onion, salt, garlic, and ginger and sauté until the onion is soft, about 5 minutes. Add the curry powder and sauté with the onion an additional 2 minutes.

3 Add the coconut milk and stir, making sure to scrape any brown bits from the bottom of the pot.

4 Add the green chilies, tomatoes, and fish pieces. Stir until well combined. Press the Cancel button. Secure the lid.

5 Press the Manual or Pressure Cook button and adjust the pressure to low and adjust the time to 5 minutes.

6 When the timer beeps, quick-release pressure until float valve drops and then unlock lid. Stir in the lemon juice and then spoon into bowls to serve.

CALORIES: 497 | **FAT**: 33g | **PROTEIN**: 39g | **SODIUM**: 982mg
FIBER: 4g | **CARBOHYDRATES**: 14g | **SUGAR**: 4g

Tomato Basil Tilapia with Quinoa

Adding quinoa to your fish dinner will make it a more filling and satisfying meal. The tomato basil salsa that tops the tilapia and quinoa in this dish adds bright flavor with a touch of sweetness. This recipe is perfect for summer when tomatoes and fresh basil are at their peak and have the best flavor.

- **Hands-On Time: 10 minutes**
- **Cook Time: 2 minutes**

Serves 4

1 cup dry quinoa
1 cup chicken stock
4 (4-ounce) tilapia filets
½ teaspoon salt, divided
¼ teaspoon black pepper, divided
3 Roma tomatoes, cored and roughly chopped
2 cloves garlic, minced
5 large fresh basil leaves, chiffonade
2 tablespoons extra-virgin olive oil

1 Add the quinoa and stock to the inner pot and place the steam rack on top. Place the tilapia on top of the steam rack and season the filets with ¼ teaspoon salt and ⅛ teaspoon pepper. Secure the lid.

2 Press the Manual or Pressure Cook button and adjust the time to 2 minutes.

3 While the Instant Pot® is coming to pressure and cooking, combine the tomatoes, garlic, basil, and oil in a small bowl. Set aside.

4 When the timer beeps, let pressure release naturally until float valve drops and then unlock lid.

5 Remove the rack and tilapia from the pot. Use a fork to fluff the quinoa, and then divide it among four plates. Place one tilapia filet on top of the quinoa, and then add the tomato mixture on top of the fish and quinoa.

CALORIES: 376 | **FAT**: 12g | **PROTEIN**: 32g | **SODIUM**: 441mg
FIBER: 6g | **CARBOHYDRATES**: 37g | **SUGAR**: 2g

Asian Chopped Kale Salad with Salmon

When you combine kale with salmon, you have a nutritional powerhouse meal. This can be an extremely quick meal; while the salmon is cooking in the Instant Pot®, chop the kale and the rest of the vegetables and prepare your dressing. When the timer beeps, all you'll need to do is add the salmon to your salad and dinner is served!

- **Hands-On Time: 20 minutes**
- **Cook Time: 3 minutes**

Serves 4

1 pound salmon
1 teaspoon salt, divided
½ teaspoon black pepper, divided
1 tablespoon lemon juice
2 bunches kale (about 12 ounces total), deveined and finely chopped
1 medium red bell pepper, seeded and diced
1 cup diced carrot
3 cups chopped cabbage
¼ cup pure sesame oil
¼ cup almond butter
¼ cup raw honey
Juice from 2 medium limes
1 tablespoon reduced sodium tamari
¼ teaspoon minced garlic
⅓ cup sesame seeds

1 Season the salmon with ½ teaspoon salt, ¼ teaspoon pepper, and the lemon juice.

2 Place 1 cup water in the inner pot of the Instant Pot® and place the steam rack inside. Place the salmon on top of the steam rack. Secure the lid.

3 Press the Manual or Pressure Cook button and adjust the time to 3 minutes.

4 When the timer beeps, let pressure release naturally until float valve drops and then unlock lid.

5 Remove the salmon from the Instant Pot® and allow it to cool completely. Once it is cool, cut it into bite-sized pieces.

6 In a large bowl, mix together the kale, bell peppers, carrots, and cabbage. Top with the salmon.

7 In a small blender, blend together the oil, almond butter, honey, lime juice, tamari, and garlic until smooth.

8 Pour the dressing onto the kale salad and toss to coat. Add the sesame seeds and lightly toss. Top with the remaining salt and pepper.

CALORIES: 579 | **FAT**: 30g | **PROTEIN**: 34g | **SODIUM**: 844mg
FIBER: 9g | **CARBOHYDRATES**: 41g | **SUGAR**: 25g

Salmon with Red Potatoes and Spinach

There's not much better than being able to cook your entire dinner in one pot. The amazing Instant Pot® makes that possible, and this salmon dinner might just become a new family favorite. The garlicky potatoes and greens are full of tremendous flavor and are two anti-inflammatory superstars!

- **Hands-On Time: 10 minutes**
- **Cook Time: 7 minutes**

Serves 4

1 pound small red potatoes, quartered
1 cup water
1¼ teaspoons salt, divided
¾ teaspoon black pepper, divided
4 (5-ounce) salmon filets
¼ teaspoon sweet paprika
½ teaspoon lemon zest
4 cloves garlic, minced
2 tablespoons avocado oil
4 cups packed baby spinach
4 lemon wedges

1 Place the potatoes in the inner pot and add 1 cup water, ¼ teaspoon salt, and ¼ teaspoon pepper. Place a steam rack on top of the potatoes.

2 On top of the salmon add the paprika, lemon zest, ½ teaspoon salt, and ¼ teaspoon pepper and place the salmon on top of the steam rack. Secure the lid.

3 Press the Manual or Pressure Cook button and adjust the time to 3 minutes.

4 When the timer beeps, let pressure release naturally until float valve drops and then unlock lid.

5 Remove the salmon and steam rack from the pot and set aside.

6 Press the Sauté button and cook the potatoes 1 minute. Add the garlic and cook an additional 2 minutes, stirring frequently. Stir in the oil and the remaining salt and pepper. Use a fork to gently mash the potatoes to achieve a chunky texture. Press the Cancel button.

7 Add the spinach and stir until wilted, about 1–2 minutes. Serve the salmon and potato and spinach mixture with the lemon wedges.

CALORIES: 332 | **FAT**: 11g | **PROTEIN**: 32g | **SODIUM**: 877mg
FIBER: 3g | **CARBOHYDRATES**: 20g | **SUGAR**: 2g

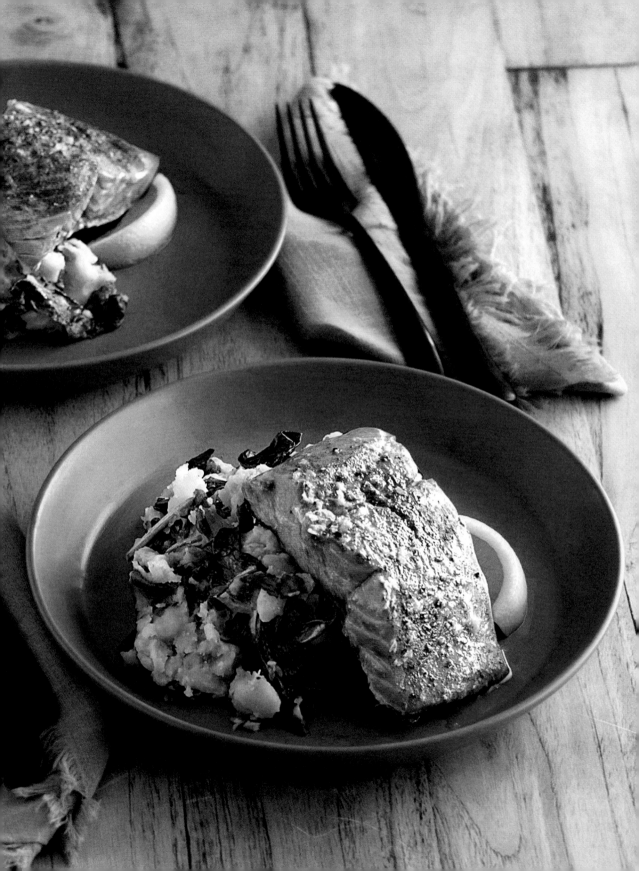

Orange Ginger Salmon

When you take a few minutes to let your salmon marinate before cooking, the results are worth the time and effort. Orange and ginger come together to create a deliciously flavored fish that will make you want more. This dish pairs perfectly wish Steamed Broccoli and Saucy Brussels Sprouts and Carrots (see recipes in Chapter 6).

- **Hands-On Time: 35 minutes**
- **Cook Time: 3 minutes**

Serves 4

1 teaspoon peeled and grated fresh ginger

2 cloves garlic, minced

1 tablespoon coconut aminos

1 tablespoon fresh orange juice

1 tablespoon almond butter

½ teaspoon salt

1 pound salmon

THE POWER OF FRESH GINGER

In addition to its anti-inflammatory benefits, fresh ginger is also often used to treat nausea and morning sickness. Food is medicine!

1   In a blender, place the ginger, garlic, coconut aminos, orange juice, almond butter, and salt and blend until smooth.

2   Place the salmon into a 7-cup glass bowl and pour the marinade over the salmon. Place this in the refrigerator and allow to marinate 30 minutes.

3   Add 1 cup water to the inner pot and place the steam rack inside. Place the bowl with the salmon on top of the steam rack. Secure the lid.

4   Press the Manual or Pressure Cook button and adjust the time to 3 minutes.

5   When the timer beeps, let pressure release naturally until float valve drops and then unlock lid. Remove the salmon from the bowl and serve.

CALORIES: 176 | **FAT**: 5g | **PROTEIN**: 24g | **SODIUM**: 460mg
FIBER: 0g | **CARBOHYDRATES**: 2g | **SUGAR**: 1g

Lemony Salmon and Asparagus

With the nutrition salmon offers, it's great to have a variety of recipes for including it in your diet on a regular basis. This is the perfect dish to serve in the spring, when asparagus is in season and inexpensive to buy. You will love the way everything cooks in one pot and dinner is ready faster than ever!

- **Hands-On Time: 5 minutes**
- **Cook Time: 3 minutes**

Serves 2

1 medium lemon
2 (5-ounce) salmon filets
2 tablespoons avocado oil, divided
½ teaspoon salt, divided
¼ teaspoon black pepper, divided
10 large asparagus spears, woody ends removed

1 Zest the lemon and set the zest aside. Slice half of the lemon and juice the other half.

2 Brush each salmon filet with ½ tablespoon avocado oil, then top with ⅛ teaspoon salt and 1/16 teaspoon pepper.

3 Add the remaining oil, salt, and pepper to the asparagus spears.

4 Place the salmon and asparagus in a steamer basket. Pour the lemon juice on top of the salmon and asparagus and sprinkle with the zest.

5 Place 1 cup water in the inner pot and place the steam rack inside. Place the steamer basket with the salmon and asparagus on top of the rack. Secure the lid.

6 Press the Manual or Pressure Cook button and adjust the time to 3 minutes.

7 When the timer beeps, let pressure release naturally until float valve drops and then unlock lid.

CALORIES: 326 | **FAT**: 18g | **PROTEIN**: 31g | **SODIUM**: 689mg
FIBER: 3g | **CARBOHYDRATES**: 5g | **SUGAR**: 2g

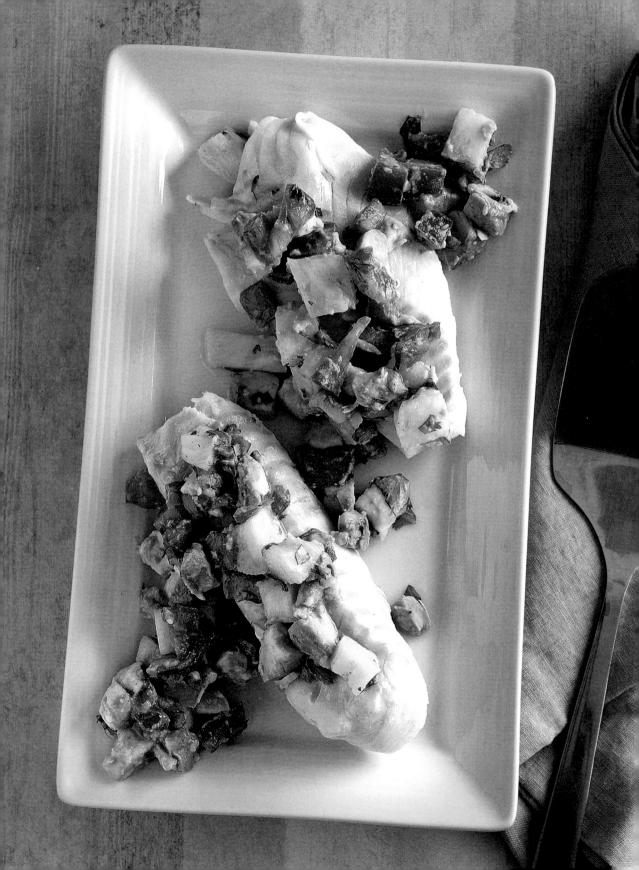

Halibut with Pineapple Avocado Salsa

Simple halibut is treated with a creamy, sweet and spicy Pineapple Avocado Salsa for a flavorful and beautiful contrast to its mild taste. Bromelain, the mixture of enzymes present in pineapple, make it a strong anti-inflammatory food so don't skip the pineapple salsa in this dish! Serve this dinner with a vegetable side of your choice and either rice or quinoa for a well-rounded, satisfying meal.

- **Hands-On Time: 15 minutes**
- **Cook Time: 3 minutes**

Serves 4

2 medium avocados, peeled, pitted, and diced

1 cup diced pineapple

2 medium tomatoes, seeded and diced

1 medium jalapeño pepper, seeded and diced

½ cup chopped cilantro

1 medium lime, juiced

1 teaspoon salt, divided

⅛ teaspoon cayenne pepper

4 (4-ounce) halibut filets

¼ teaspoon black pepper

DOUBLE UP

You're going to love this Pineapple Avocado Salsa so much, you should make a double batch so you also have some for snacking.

1 In a medium bowl, combine the avocado, pineapple, tomatoes, jalapeño, cilantro, lime juice, ½ teaspoon salt, and cayenne pepper. Place in the refrigerator while the halibut cooks.

2 Season the halibut with remaining ½ teaspoon salt and black pepper.

3 Place 1 cup water in the inner pot of the Instant Pot® and place the steam rack inside. Place the halibut on top of the steam rack. Secure the lid.

4 Press the Manual or Pressure Cook button and adjust the time to 3 minutes.

5 When the timer beeps, let pressure release naturally until float valve drops and then unlock lid.

6 Transfer the halibut filets to plates and top each filet with a portion of the Pineapple Avocado Salsa.

CALORIES: 250 | **FAT**: 11g | **PROTEIN**: 23g | **SODIUM**: 667mg
FIBER: 6g | **CARBOHYDRATES**: 14g | **SUGAR**: 6g

Mediterranean Salmon Salad

The Mediterranean diet has been touted as one of the world's healthiest ways of eating. When you research this diet you'll learn that it is very much in line with the anti-inflammatory diet. This salad embraces Mediterranean flavor as well as the nutrition that comes from its ingredients!

- **Hands-On Time: 20 minutes**
- **Cook Time: 3 minutes**

Serves 4

1 pound salmon
1 teaspoon salt, divided
½ teaspoon black pepper, divided
1 tablespoon lemon juice
1½ tablespoons extra-virgin olive oil
1 tablespoon fresh lemon juice
½ tablespoon apple cider vinegar
1 tablespoon chopped fresh parsley
2 teaspoons minced garlic
½ teaspoon dried oregano
4 cups chopped romaine lettuce
1 large cucumber, diced
2 Roma tomatoes, cored and diced
1 medium red onion, peeled and sliced
1 medium avocado, peeled, pitted, and sliced
⅓ cup pitted Kalamata olives, sliced

1 Season the salmon with ½ teaspoon salt, ¼ teaspoon pepper, and the lemon juice.

2 Place 1 cup water in the inner pot of the Instant Pot® and place the steam rack inside. Place the salmon on top of the steam rack. Secure the lid.

3 Press the Manual or Pressure Cook button and adjust the time to 3 minutes.

4 Meanwhile, prepare the dressing and salad ingredients. Into a small container or jar with a tight lid, place the oil, lemon juice, vinegar, parsley, garlic, oregano, ½ teaspoon salt, and ¼ teaspoon pepper. Shake well until combined and set aside.

5 Place the lettuce, cucumber, tomatoes, red onion, avocado, and olives in a large bowl. Set aside.

6 When the timer beeps, let pressure release naturally until float valve drops and then unlock lid.

7 Remove the salmon from the Instant Pot® and allow it to cool completely. Once it is cool, cut it into bite-sized pieces.

8 Add the salmon pieces to the salad bowl. Drizzle with the dressing and gently toss to combine.

CALORIES: 329 | **FAT**: 18g | **PROTEIN**: 26g | **SODIUM**: 964mg
FIBER: 5g | **CARBOHYDRATES**: 12g | **SUGAR**: 4g

Vegetarian Main Dishes

In this chapter vegetables take the center stage and get to be the star of the show and your plate. You don't have to be a vegetarian to eat vegetarian food. Even if you aren't a vegetarian, it's an excellent idea to incorporate two to four vegetarian meals into your week. Whenever you take meat off your plate, you're adding in more plant foods, which have more phytonutrients and anti-inflammatory compounds than any other food group on the planet.

If you're new to eating vegetarian meals, you are going to be amazed at how hearty and satisfying they can be. Most of them combine whole grains or beans with vegetables, all of which are full of fiber and protein along with vitamins and minerals.

From the flavorful Loaded Sweet Potatoes to the unique Spinach Artichoke Chickpea Casserole, you just might find your new favorite meal in this chapter. The Instant Pot® makes your vegetarian dinners quick and easy, and in many case in just one pot!

Broccoli Rice Casserole

In many parts of the country casseroles are a part of everyday cooking. Unfortunately, they aren't always the healthiest dinner option. This vegetarian main-course casserole is one you can feel great about feeding your family. It's got that cozy, down-home feel to it, yet it's filled with nourishing ingredients. It's a stick-to-your-ribs kind of meal that will leave you satisfied.

- **Hands-On Time: 15 minutes**
- **Cook Time: 37 minutes**

Serves 6

1 tablespoon avocado oil

1 medium yellow onion, peeled and diced

2 cloves garlic, minced

1½ cups brown rice

4 cups vegetable broth

3 cups large broccoli florets

1 (15-ounce) can cooked chickpeas, drained and rinsed

½ cup nutritional yeast

1 teaspoon paprika

½ teaspoon salt

1 Add the oil to the inner pot. Press the Sauté button and heat the oil 1 minute. Add the onion and sauté 5 minutes. Add the garlic and sauté an additional 30 seconds. Add the rice and stir to coat with the onions, oil, and garlic. Press the Cancel button.

2 Add the broth and secure the lid. Press the Manual or Pressure Cook button and then adjust the pressure to low and adjust the time to 25 minutes.

3 When the timer beeps, quick-release pressure until float valve drops and then unlock lid.

4 Add broccoli and secure the lid. Press the Manual or Pressure Cook button and then adjust the pressure to low and adjust the time to 5 minutes.

5 When the timer beeps, quick-release pressure until float valve drops and then unlock lid.

6 Stir in the chickpeas, nutritional yeast, paprika, and salt. Spoon into bowls and serve.

CALORIES: 308 | **FAT**: 4g | **PROTEIN**: 11g | **SODIUM**: 673mg
FIBER: 8g | **CARBOHYDRATES**: 55g | **SUGAR**: 4g

Lentil-Stuffed Spaghetti Squash

Lentils are high in protein and iron and are an excellent stand-in for meat in recipes like this. Here they are cooked with a number of anti-inflammatory ingredients like garlic, ginger, and turmeric. Those are just bonuses, though, because all you'll be thinking about is how flavorful and satisfying this dish is.

- **Hands-On Time: 10 minutes**
- **Cook Time: 27 minutes**

Serves 2

1 tablespoon avocado oil

1 small yellow onion, peeled and diced

1 teaspoon minced garlic

1½ teaspoons peeled and coarsely chopped fresh ginger

1 cup brown lentils

2 cups vegetable broth

1 teaspoon ground cumin

1 teaspoon turmeric

½ teaspoon kosher salt

¼ teaspoon black pepper

2 medium cooked spaghetti squash halves

TWO INSTANT POTS®?

You can use the Simple Spaghetti Squash recipe in Chapter 6 to cook your spaghetti squash ahead of time. Better yet, if you have two Instant Pots® you can cook everything at once!

1 Add the oil to the inner pot. Press the Sauté button and heat the oil 1 minute. Add the onion and sauté 5 minutes. Add the garlic and ginger and sauté an additional 30 seconds. Press the Cancel button.

2 Add the lentils, broth, cumin, turmeric, salt, and pepper and stir to combine. Secure the lid.

3 Press the Manual or Pressure Cook button and adjust the time to 20 minutes.

4 When the timer beeps, quick-release pressure until float valve drops and then unlock lid.

5 Meanwhile, scrape the spaghetti squash strands from the cooked spaghetti squash halves into a large bowl. Reserve the shells.

6 Add the lentils to the bowl with the squash and toss to combine.

7 Divide the mixture between the shells and serve.

CALORIES: 551 | FAT: 9g | PROTEIN: 28g | SODIUM: 1,174mg
FIBER: 20g | CARBOHYDRATES: 95g | SUGAR: 12g

Chickpea-Stuffed Acorn Squash

Acorn squash has a lovely, buttery flavor that pairs well with the spicy chickpeas in this recipe. Typically, it takes 30–45 minutes to cook your acorn squash in the oven, but with your Instant Pot® it cooks quickly in just 5 minutes. Acorn squash is high in beta-carotene, which helps prevent the oxidative stress caused by free radicals. This is a perfect dish to serve in the fall when acorn squash is in peak season.

- **Hands-On Time: 5 minutes**
- **Cook Time: 12 minutes**

Serves 2

1 medium acorn squash, cut in half and seeds removed
½ teaspoon salt, divided
1 tablespoon avocado oil
1 (15-ounce) can chickpeas, drained, rinsed, and dried
¼ teaspoon black pepper
½ teaspoon allspice
½ teaspoon ground ginger

1 Place ½ cup water in the inner pot of your Instant Pot® and place the steam rack inside.

2 Sprinkle the acorn squash halves with ⅛ teaspoon salt each. Place the acorn squash, cut side up, on the steam rack. Secure the lid.

3 Press the Manual or Pressure Cook button and adjust the time to 5 minutes.

4 When the timer beeps, quick-release pressure until float valve drops and then unlock lid.

5 Carefully remove the squash and place on a plate. Cover with aluminum foil to keep warm.

6 Remove the water and steam rack from the inner pot and dry the pot.

7 Press the Sauté button and then use the Adjust button to change to the More setting. Add the oil to the inner pot. Allow it to heat 2 minutes.

8 Add the chickpeas, ¼ teaspoon salt, pepper, allspice, and ginger to the inner pot and sauté until the chickpeas are lightly browned, about 5 minutes. Press the Cancel button.

9 Remove the chickpeas from the inner pot and add half to each of the cooked acorn squash shells. Serve immediately.

CALORIES: 335 | **FAT**: 9g | **PROTEIN**: 11g | **SODIUM**: 868mg
FIBER: 12g | **CARBOHYDRATES**: 54g | **SUGAR**: 5g

Loaded Sweet Potatoes

Can a sweet potato be a main dish? When it's loaded with a tasty filling of beans it absolutely can! These Loaded Sweet Potatoes have Mexican-inspired flavors and are incredibly filling. Nobody is going to complain about being unsatisfied after this meal. The Instant Pot® makes it easy to cook the bean filling and the sweet potatoes at the same time!

- **Hands-On Time: 10 minutes**
- **Cook Time: 26 minutes**

Serves 2

1½ tablespoons avocado oil

1 small white onion, peeled and diced

3 cloves garlic, minced

1 teaspoon ground cumin

1 teaspoon ground chili powder

½ teaspoon kosher salt

½ teaspoon dried oregano

¼ teaspoon black pepper

¼ pound dry pinto beans

1½ cups vegetable broth

2 medium sweet potatoes

1   Add the oil to the inner pot. Press the Sauté button and heat the oil 1 minute. Add the onion and sauté until starting to brown, about 6–7 minutes. Add the garlic, cumin, chili powder, salt, oregano, and pepper and sauté an additional 1 minute. Press the Cancel button.

2   Add the beans and broth to the inner pot. Place the steam rack inside and place the sweet potatoes on top of the rack. Secure the lid.

3   Press the Manual or Pressure Cook button and adjust the time to 18 minutes.

4   When the timer beeps, quick-release pressure until float valve drops and then unlock lid.

5   To serve, cut each sweet potato in half and top with half of the bean mixture.

CALORIES: 440 | FAT: 11g | PROTEIN: 15g | SODIUM: 1,105mg
FIBER: 15g | CARBOHYDRATES: 70g | SUGAR: 9g

Quinoa Burrito Bowls

Sometimes plant-based meals get a bad rep for being too light or unsatisfying, but that's just not true. You don't always have to add animal protein to your meals when you are eating high-quality protein plant foods like beans and quinoa. Nothing is lacking in this flavorful, bright burrito bowl.

- **Hands-On Time: 5 minutes**
- **Cook Time: 10 minutes**

Serves 4

2 teaspoons avocado oil
½ medium red onion, peeled and diced
1 medium red bell pepper, seeded and diced
½ teaspoon salt
1 teaspoon cumin
1 teaspoon minced garlic
1 cup quinoa
1 cup no-sugar-added, low sodium salsa
1 cup vegetable stock
1 (15-ounce) can black beans, drained and rinsed
1 medium avocado, peeled pitted and sliced
1 cup chopped fresh cilantro
1 scallion, sliced
1 medium lime, cut into 4 wedges

1 Press the Sauté button and add the oil to the inner pot. Add the onion, bell pepper, salt, and cumin and cook 5 minutes. Add the garlic and cook another 30 seconds. Press the Cancel button.

2 Add the quinoa, salsa, stock, and beans and stir to combine, scraping up any brown bits that may be stuck to the bottom of the pot. Secure the lid.

3 Press the Manual or Pressure Cook button and adjust the time to 5 minutes.

4 When the timer beeps, let pressure release naturally until float valve drops and then unlock lid.

5 Spoon the quinoa mixture into four bowls and top with the avocado, cilantro, and scallions. Serve with the lime wedges.

CALORIES: 371 | FAT: 10g | PROTEIN: 14g | SODIUM: 773mg
FIBER: 14g | CARBOHYDRATES: 56g | SUGAR: 5g

Root Vegetable Lentil Bowls

Root vegetables and lentils come together to create a cozy, down-home dish that is a stick-to-your-ribs kind of dinner. Sautéing the vegetables and garlic before cooking with the lentils adds a nice depth of flavor to the final dish.

- **Hands-On Time: 10 minutes**
- **Cook Time: 26 minutes**

Serves 4

1 tablespoon avocado oil
1 medium yellow onion, peeled and chopped
6 cloves garlic, minced
1 large carrot, peeled and chopped
1 large parsnip, peeled and chopped
1 small turnip, peeled and chopped
2 medium stalks celery, ends removed and sliced
1 teaspoon salt
1 teaspoon dried thyme
1 teaspoon dried oregano
¼ teaspoon black pepper
1 cup brown lentils
2½ cups vegetable stock

1 Pour the oil into the inner pot. Press the Sauté button. Add the onion and cook 5 minutes, stirring occasionally.

2 Add the garlic, carrot, parsnip, turnip, celery, salt, thyme, oregano, and black pepper. Stir to combine and cook another 30 seconds. Press the Cancel button.

3 Add the lentils and stir to combine, then add the stock. Secure the lid.

4 Press the Manual or Pressure Cook button and adjust the time to 20 minutes.

5 When the timer beeps, quick-release pressure until float valve drops and then unlock lid. Spoon into bowls and serve.

CALORIES: 268 | **FAT**: 5g | **PROTEIN**: 17g | **SODIUM**: 1,167mg
FIBER: 9g | **CARBOHYDRATES**: 45g | **SUGAR**: 6g

CAN YOU SUBSTITUTE ANOTHER KIND OF LENTIL?
It's important to stick to brown lentils in this recipe because the cooking time varies a lot among different lentil varieties. Red lentils, for example, would completely disintegrate in 20 minutes in the Instant Pot®.

Spinach Artichoke Chickpea Casserole

Spinach and artichokes are a classic combination, and they come together once again for this charming vegetarian dinner. Lemon juice and lemon zest brighten the entire dish, and you'll love the contrasting textures with the chickpeas. Casseroles typically take 30 minutes to bake in the oven, but with the Instant Pot® the cook time is only 6 minutes!

- **Hands-On Time: 7 minutes**
- **Cook Time: 6 minutes**

Serves 2

1 tablespoon avocado oil

1 medium yellow onion, peeled and finely chopped

2 cloves garlic, minced

1 (15.5-ounce) can chickpeas, drained and dried

1 (14-ounce) can baby artichokes, drained and roughly chopped

½ cup vegetable stock

1 tablespoon fresh lemon juice

1 tablespoon fresh thyme leaves

1 teaspoon lemon zest

2½ ounces baby spinach

1 Press the Sauté button and pour the oil into the inner pot. After it heats 1 minute, add the onion. Allow it to cook, stirring occasionally, 3 minutes.

2 Add the garlic and chickpeas, stir to combine, and cook 1 more minute. Press the Cancel button.

3 Add the artichokes and stock. Secure the lid.

4 Press the Manual or Pressure Cook button and adjust the time to 1 minute.

5 When the timer beeps, quick-release pressure until float valve drops and then unlock lid.

6 Stir in the lemon juice, thyme leaves, lemon zest, and half of the baby spinach. Stir until well combined and then add the rest of the spinach. Continue to stir until all of the spinach leaves are wilted. Transfer to bowls and serve.

CALORIES: 352 | **FAT**: 8g | **PROTEIN**: 15g | **SODIUM**: 871mg
FIBER: 17g | **CARBOHYDRATES**: 52g | **SUGAR**: 9g

Sweet Potato Chickpea Hash

Chickpeas do a great job taking the place of meat in this one-bowl meal. One thing that chickpeas add to this dish that turkey cannot is fiber! This is going to help you with digestion, and a diet high in fiber is also important for maintaining healthy cholesterol levels and preventing heart disease and diabetes. This recipe makes it easy to switch out the meat in favor of a plant-based alternative.

- **Hands-On Time: 10 minutes**
- **Cook Time: 12 minutes**

Serves 2

1½ tablespoons avocado oil

1 medium yellow onion, peeled and diced

2 cloves garlic, minced

1 cup vegetable stock

1 medium sweet potato, cut into cubes (peeling not necessary)

1 (15-ounce) can chickpeas, drained and rinsed

½ teaspoon salt

1 teaspoon Italian seasoning blend

½ cup chopped flat-leaf parsley

1 Press the Sauté button and add the oil. Allow the oil to heat 1 minute and then add the onion and cook until softened, about 5 minutes. Add the garlic and cook an additional 30 seconds. Press the Cancel button.

2 Add stock, sweet potato, chickpeas, salt, and Italian seasoning and stir to combine. Secure the lid.

3 Press the Manual or Pressure Cook button and adjust the time to 5 minutes.

4 When the timer beeps, quick-release pressure until float valve drops and then unlock lid.

5 Spoon the mixture into bowls and top with the parsley.

CALORIES: 370 | **FAT**: 13g | **PROTEIN**: 13g | **SODIUM**: 1,340mg
FIBER: 12g | **CARBOHYDRATES**: 51g | **SUGAR**: 11g

Coconut Curry Lentil Chickpea Bowls with Kale

If there is such a thing as "healthy comfort food," this dish definitely qualifies. It's a dish that will make you feel happy when you're eating it, enjoying the warming spices and creamy texture. Of course, the ease of preparation makes it even more attractive! This recipe is sure to make it into your regular rotation.

- **Hands-On Time: 10 minutes**
- **Cook Time: 8 minutes**

Serves 4

¾ cup red lentils

1 (15-ounce) can diced tomatoes with garlic and onion, with juices

1 (13.66-ounce) can unsweetened lite coconut milk

1 cup vegetable broth

1 tablespoon curry powder

1 teaspoon peeled and grated fresh ginger

1 teaspoon turmeric

1 teaspoon salt

1 (15-ounce) can chickpeas, drained and rinsed

4 cups finely chopped, deveined kale

1 tablespoon lime juice

⅓ cup roughly chopped fresh cilantro leaves and stems

1 Place all of the ingredients, except the kale, lime juice, and cilantro leaves, in the inner pot and stir to combine well. Secure the lid.

2 Press the Manual or Pressure Cook button and adjust the time to 8 minutes.

3 When the timer beeps, let pressure release naturally until float valve drops and then unlock lid.

4 Stir in the kale and lime juice. Spoon into bowls and serve topped with cilantro.

CALORIES: 328 | FAT: 8g | PROTEIN: 15g | SODIUM: 1,066mg
FIBER: 12g | CARBOHYDRATES: 48g | SUGAR: 6g

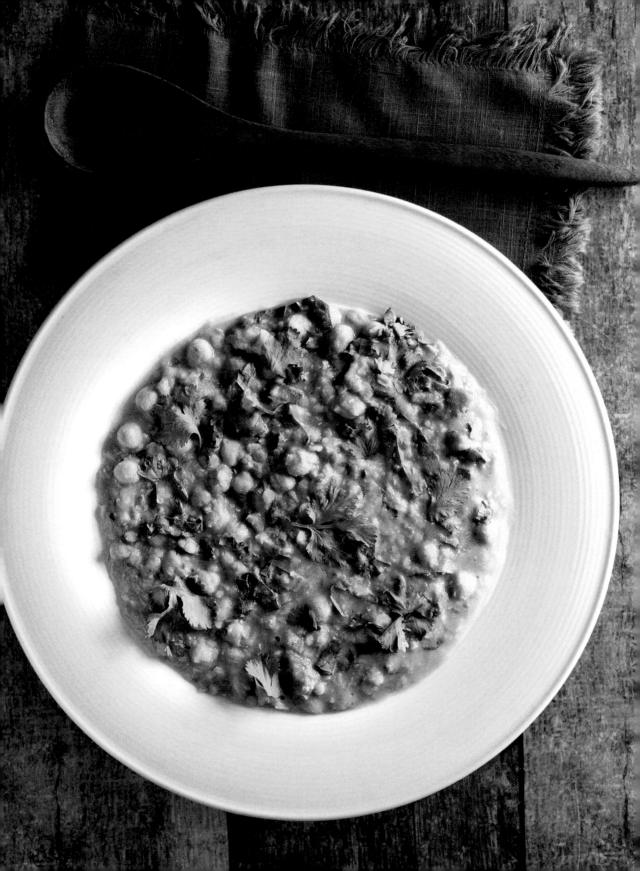

Vegetable Rice and Beans with Turmeric

Rice and beans get a major upgrade by adding in a healthy dose of vegetables and anti-inflammatory powerhouse turmeric. The flavor of fresh turmeric is quite different than its dried counterpart, and it's something you need to experience. Due to its recent rise to the spotlight, you can find fresh turmeric root in the produce section of most well-stocked supermarkets.

- **Hands-On Time: 10 minutes**
- **Cook Time: 44 minutes**

Serves 4

1 tablespoon avocado oil

1 small yellow onion, peeled and diced

2 medium carrots, peeled, ends removed and chopped

2 medium stalks celery, ends removed and chopped

2 teaspoons peeled and chopped fresh turmeric

¼ teaspoon salt

⅛ teaspoon black pepper

1 cup long grain brown basmati rice

1⅓ cups vegetable stock

1 (15-ounce) can red kidney beans, drained and rinsed

1 cup chopped fresh parsley

1　Pour the oil into the inner pot and press the Sauté button. Allow the oil to heat 1 minute and then add the onion, carrots, and celery. Cook 5 minutes, stirring occasionally.

2　Add the turmeric, salt, pepper, and rice and sauté, stirring frequently, another 5 minutes.

3　Add the stock and use a wooden spoon to scrape up any brown bits from the bottom of the Instant Pot®. Press the Cancel button. Secure the lid.

4　Press the Manual or Pressure Cook button and adjust the time to 33 minutes.

5　When the timer beeps, let pressure release naturally until float valve drops and then unlock lid.

6　While the Instant Pot® is still in Keep Warm mode, stir in the beans.

7　Divide the rice and bean mixture among four plates and top each with ¼ cup fresh parsley.

CALORIES: 320 | FAT: 6g | PROTEIN: 11g | SODIUM: 771mg
FIBER: 9g | CARBOHYDRATES: 57g | SUGAR: 3g

Kale Power Bowls

If you think kale is too bitter for your taste buds, this recipe could change your mind. When mixed with a tangy dressing made with fresh lemon juice, tahini, and garlic, the kale becomes more mellow. Buckwheat groats and butternut squash bring their own nutty and sweet flavor to this hearty vegetarian meal.

- **Hands-On Time: 10 minutes**
- **Cook Time: 5 minutes**

Serves 4

¾ cup buckwheat groats

1¾ cups vegetable broth

1 (10-ounce) bag frozen butternut squash cubes

¼ cup fresh lemon juice

¼ cup tahini

1 clove garlic

3 tablespoons nutritional yeast

3 tablespoons water

1 teaspoon Dijon mustard

1 medium bunch red kale, stems removed and finely chopped (about 6 ounces)

¼ teaspoon salt

¼ teaspoon black pepper

1 Place the buckwheat groats, broth, and squash in the inner pot. Secure the lid.

2 Press the Manual or Pressure Cook button and adjust the time to 5 minutes.

3 Meanwhile, in a blender, place the lemon juice, tahini, garlic, nutritional yeast, water, and mustard and blend until smooth. Set aside.

4 When the timer beeps, quick-release pressure until float valve drops and then unlock lid.

5 Place the chopped kale in a medium bowl. Top with the butternut squash and buckwheat groats and toss to combine. Add the lemon-tahini dressing, salt, and pepper, and toss again to coat. Serve warm.

CALORIES: 277 | FAT: 8g | PROTEIN: 11g | SODIUM: 448mg
FIBER: 8g | CARBOHYDRATES: 45g | SUGAR: 4g

CHOP CHOP!
Pay attention to the recipe instructions to chop the kale finely as it makes a difference in the final result of this dish. Finely chopped kale will be able to soften slightly when mixed with the hot portion of this recipe, and it makes it more tender and easy to chew.

Autumn Harvest Quinoa Bowl

This has all of the flavors of autumn in one amazing bowl. Quinoa and white beans provide protein and the butternut squash's soft texture is balanced by the crunch of chopped walnuts. The dressing delivers irresistible flavor. Look for fruit juice–sweetened dried cranberries as regular dried cranberries can be loaded with refined sugar.

- **Hands-On Time: 10 minutes**
- **Cook Time: 5 minutes**

Serves 4

6 tablespoons extra-virgin olive oil

3 tablespoons apple cider vinegar

½ teaspoon Dijon mustard

½ teaspoon minced garlic

½ teaspoon dried thyme

½ teaspoon dried rosemary

½ teaspoon salt

¼ teaspoon black pepper

1 cup quinoa

1¼ cups vegetable stock

1 (10-ounce) bag frozen butternut squash cubes

1 (15-ounce) can cannelloni beans, drained and rinsed

4 cups baby kale leaves

½ cup fruit-juice sweetened dried cranberries

½ cup chopped walnuts

½ cup chopped fresh parsley

SUBSTITUTION SUGGESTION

If you are unable to find fruit juice–sweetened dried cranberries, look for unsweetened dried tart cherries or raisins as an acceptable substitution.

1 In a small jar or container with a tight lid, place the oil, vinegar, mustard, garlic, thyme, rosemary, salt, and pepper and shake until well combined. Set aside.

2 Place the quinoa, stock, frozen butternut squash cubes, and beans into the inner pot and stir to combine. Secure the lid.

3 Press the Manual or Pressure Cook button and adjust the time to 5 minutes.

4 When the timer beeps, quick-release pressure until float valve drops and then unlock lid.

5 Stir in the kale leaves until they are wilted. Spoon the quinoa mixture into four bowls and top with the dried cranberries, walnuts, and fresh parsley. Drizzle each bowl with one quarter of the dressing and toss to combine.

CALORIES: 609 | **FAT**: 32g | **PROTEIN**: 16g | **SODIUM**: 773mg
FIBER: 13g | **CARBOHYDRATES**: 70g | **SUGAR**: 12g

Avocado Egg Salad with Arugula

While over the years there's been a lot of disagreements about whether or not eggs are a healthy food, no one can argue with the nutrients they contain. Eggs are an excellent source of protein, fat-soluble vitamins, essential fatty acids, and a wide range of minerals like iron, calcium, manganese, and selenium. And before you let your yolk go down the drain, remember that the majority of these nutrients are concentrated in that little yellow center. This recipe gives you a simple and delicious way to enjoy your eggs.

- **Hands-On Time: 10 minutes**
- **Cook Time: 7 minutes**

Serves 2

3 large eggs
1 small avocado, peeled, pitted, and mashed
1 teaspoon Dijon mustard
1 tablespoon apple cider vinegar
¼ teaspoon garlic powder
¼ teaspoon dried dill weed
¼ teaspoon salt
1 tablespoon flat-leaf parsley, chopped
2 cups baby arugula leaves

1 Pour 1 cup water into the inner pot of your Instant Pot® and place the steam rack inside.

2 Carefully place eggs directly onto the steam rack.

3 Press the Steam button and adjust the time to 7 minutes.

4 When the timer beeps, quick-release pressure until float valve drops and then unlock lid.

5 Immediately transfer the eggs to a bowl filled with iced water and let them sit for 15 minutes.

6 Remove the eggs from the water and peel the shell away from the eggs.

7 Roughly chop the eggs and add them to a medium bowl. Add the avocado, mustard, vinegar, garlic powder, dill weed, salt, and parsley and stir to combine.

8 Serve on top of arugula leaves.

CALORIES: 233 | **FAT**: 16g | **PROTEIN**: 12g | **SODIUM**: 470mg
FIBER: 5g | **CARBOHYDRATES**: 8g | **SUGAR**: 1g

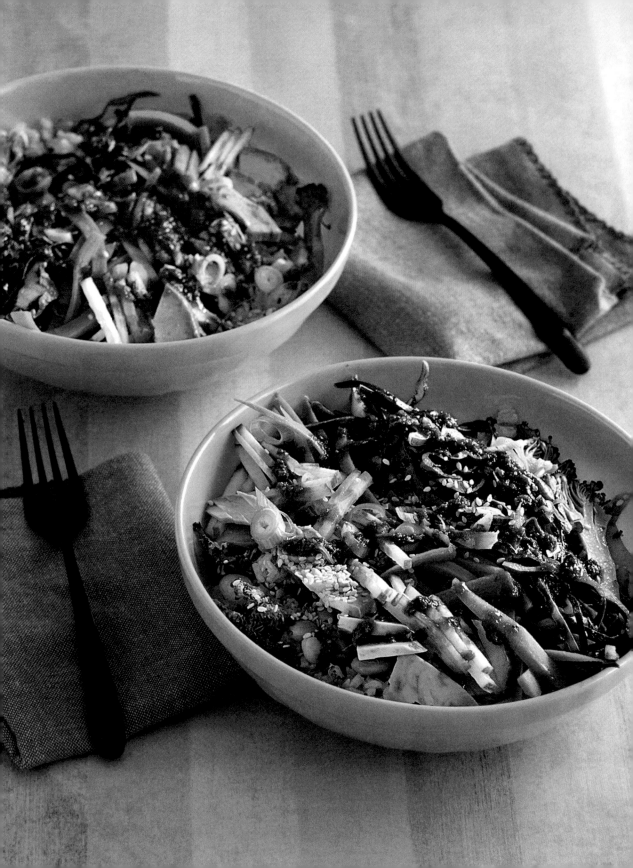

Vegetable Buddha Bowls with Carrot Ginger Dressing

"Buddha bowl" is a name for an entire meal, usually vegan, in a bowl. Buddha bowls often start with a grain, have a plant protein of some kind, and lots and lots of vegetables. The Carrot Ginger Dressing in this bowl is not only a delicious and vibrant dressing, it also has powerful anti-inflammatory powers thanks to both the ginger and carrots!

- **Hands-On Time: 20 minutes**
- **Cook Time: 26 minutes**

Serves 4

1 cup short-grain brown rice

1¼ cups vegetable stock, divided

2½ tablespoons extra-virgin olive oil

2½ tablespoons apple cider vinegar

2 large carrots, peeled and thinly sliced, divided

1 tablespoon peeled and chopped fresh ginger

1 tablespoon fresh lime juice

¼ teaspoon pure stevia powder

¾ teaspoon toasted sesame oil

⅛ teaspoon salt

1½ cups frozen shelled edamame, thawed

1½ cups thinly sliced broccoli florets

4 cups thinly sliced red cabbage

1 medium cucumber, thinly sliced

2 medium avocados, peeled, pitted, and thinly sliced

2 tablespoons sesame seeds

2 scallions, thinly sliced

1. Place the rice and 1 cup stock in the inner pot. Secure the lid.

2. Press the Manual or Pressure Cook button and adjust the time to 24 minutes.

3. While the rice is cooking, make the dressing. In a powerful blender, blend the olive oil, vinegar, half of the carrot slices, ginger, lime juice, stevia, sesame oil, and salt until the mixture is super smooth. Set aside.

4. When the timer beeps, let pressure release naturally until float valve drops and then unlock lid. Use a fork to fluff the rice. Press the Cancel button.

5. Press the Sauté button and add ¼ cup stock with the edamame and broccoli. Gently stir and then let them cook until warm, about 2 minutes.

6. To assemble the Vegetable Buddha Bowls, spoon one quarter of the rice mixture into each of the four bowls. Add one quarter each of the remaining carrot slices, cabbage, cucumber, and avocado slices to each bowl, keeping the ingredients separated. Sprinkle one quarter of the sesame seeds and scallions over each bowl and drizzle with one quarter of the Carrot Ginger Dressing.

CALORIES: 462 | **FAT:** 17g | **PROTEIN:** 17g | **SODIUM:** 400mg
FIBER: 15g | **CARBOHYDRATES:** 64g | **SUGAR:** 8g

Mexican Chopped Salad with Spicy Avocado Dressing

Who knew a vegan salad could be so hearty and filling that it's a main course? That is definitely the case with this flavorful salad. Creamy avocado gives a lovely texture to the dressing, and hot sauce gives it a little kick!

- **Hands-On Time: 15 minutes**
- **Cook Time: 15 minutes**

Serves 4

¼ pound dry black beans

1 cup water

1 small ripe avocado, peeled, pitted, and chopped

1 tablespoon extra-virgin olive oil

¾ cup chopped cilantro, divided

Juice from 2 medium limes

⅛ teaspoon fine sea salt

1 teaspoon minced garlic

¼ teaspoon hot sauce

3–5 tablespoons water

2 hearts romaine lettuce, finely chopped

1 medium red bell pepper, seeded and chopped

1 cup grape tomatoes, cut into eighths

1 scallion, green part sliced

½ teaspoon coarse salt

¼ teaspoon freshly cracked black pepper

1 Place the black beans in a large bowl and cover with 3" water. Soak the beans 4–8 hours. Drain the beans.

2 Place the soaked beans and 1 cup water in the inner pot. Secure the lid.

3 Press the Manual or Pressure Cook button and adjust the time to 15 minutes.

4 Meanwhile, prepare the Spicy Avocado Dressing. In a blender, place the avocado, olive oil, ¼ cup cilantro, lime juice, fine sea salt, garlic, and hot sauce and blend until smooth. Add enough water to create the consistency you desire. Set aside.

5 When the timer beeps, let pressure release naturally until float valve drops and then unlock lid.

6 In a large bowl, place the remaining cilantro, romaine lettuce, bell pepper, tomatoes, and scallion. Add the cooked black beans and drizzle with the dressing. Toss to coat. Top with the coarse salt and pepper and serve.

CALORIES: 250 | FAT: 12g | PROTEIN: 9g | SODIUM: 259mg
FIBER: 11g | CARBOHYDRATES: 29g | SUGAR: 4g

Loaded Spinach Salad with Creamy Avocado Dressing

Once again avocado lends its creamy texture to an amazing salad loaded with chickpeas and quinoa. The flavor is bursting with fresh basil as the star, and a hint of lemon keeps it bright and fresh. The chickpeas get a crispy texture when browned using the Sauté function on your Instant Pot®, giving this salad a great contrasting texture.

- **Hands-On Time: 7 minutes**
- **Cook Time: 11 minutes**

Serves 4

½ cup dry quinoa

1 cup vegetable stock

1 tablespoon avocado oil

1 (15-ounce) can chickpeas, drained and rinsed

¾ teaspoon salt, divided

1 medium ripe avocado

5 whole basil leaves

1 clove garlic, minced

2 tablespoons lemon juice

¼–¾ cup water

5 ounces baby spinach leaves

1 large tomato, cored, seeded, and cut into chunks

¼ teaspoon freshly ground black pepper

1 Place the quinoa in a fine-mesh strainer and rinse under water until the water runs clear.

2 Place the quinoa and stock in the inner pot. Secure the lid.

3 Press the Manual or Pressure Cook button and adjust the time to 1 minute.

4 When the timer beeps, quick-release pressure until float valve drops and then unlock lid.

5 Transfer the quinoa to a medium bowl to cool.

6 Wipe the inner pot clean and add the oil. Press the Sauté button and use the Adjust button to change the setting to More.

7 Add the chickpeas and ¼ teaspoon salt to the inner pot and cook, stirring occasionally until the chickpeas are browned and getting crispy, about 10 minutes. Press the Cancel button.

8 Meanwhile, make the dressing. Put the avocado, basil, garlic, lemon juice, ¼ teaspoon salt, and ¼ cup water in a blender and blend until smooth. Add more water, as needed, to achieve your desired consistency.

9 In a large bowl, place the spinach, tomato, quinoa, and chickpeas and then drizzle with the dressing. Toss to coat and then top with the ¼ teaspoon salt and pepper.

CALORIES: 280 | FAT: 11g | PROTEIN: 10g | SODIUM: 826mg
FIBER: 9g | CARBOHYDRATES: 36g | SUGAR: 4g

Mediterranean Sweet Potatoes

The sweet potato is a perfect base for a complete vegan meal. Topped with crispy chickpeas, tomatoes, olives, and parsley and then drizzled with a flavorful tahini-herb dressing, it's sure to knock your socks off!

- **Hands-On Time: 5 minutes**
- **Cook Time: 29 minutes**

Serves 4

4 medium sweet potatoes
¼ cup tahini
Juice of 1 medium lemon
1 tablespoon apple cider vinegar
2 cloves garlic
¼ cup fresh basil
1 teaspoon fresh oregano
1 teaspoon fresh thyme leaves
½ teaspoon salt, divided
¼ teaspoon pepper, divided
3–5 tablespoons water
1 tablespoon avocado oil
1 (15-ounce) can chickpeas, drained, rinsed, and dried
½ cup sliced black olives
½ cup sliced grape tomatoes
½ cup chopped fresh flat-leaf parsley

1 Pour 1½ cups water into your Instant Pot® and place the steam rack inside.

2 Place the sweet potatoes on the rack. It's okay if they overlap. Secure the lid.

3 Press the Manual or Pressure Cook button and adjust the time to 18 minutes.

4 Make the dressing. In a blender, combine the tahini, lemon juice, vinegar, garlic, basil, oregano, thyme, ¼ teaspoon salt, and ⅛ teaspoon pepper and blend until smooth. Add the water, 1 tablespoon at a time, as needed until desired consistency is reached. Set aside.

5 When the timer beeps, quick-release pressure until float valve drops and then unlock lid.

6 Remove sweet potatoes, place on a plate, and cover with aluminum foil to keep warm.

7 Remove the rack and water from the inner pot and dry it.

8 Press the Sauté button and use the Adjust button to change the setting to More. Add the oil and let it heat 1 minute.

9 Add the chickpeas and remaining ¼ teaspoon salt and ⅛ teaspoon pepper to the inner pot. Sauté, stirring frequently until the chickpeas are browned and crisp, about 10 minutes. Press the Cancel button.

10 Cut the sweet potatoes in half and top with one quarter of the chickpeas, olives, tomatoes, and parsley. Drizzle with the dressing.

CALORIES: 258 | **FAT**: 12g | **PROTEIN**: 5g | **SODIUM**: 502mg
FIBER: 7g | **CARBOHYDRATES**: 34g | **SUGAR**: 6g

Hearty Vegetable Rice Casserole

Brussels sprouts and carrots pair with jasmine rice for a hearty and filling meal. Cooked all together in a mouthwatering sauce, the Instant Pot® is the perfect cooking vessel for this easy dinner. Being able to sauté the vegetables and cook the rice in the same pot really cuts down on your cleanup time.

- **Hands-On Time: 15 minutes**
- **Cook Time: 8 minutes**

Serves 4

1 cup vegetable broth
¼ cup fresh lime juice
¼ cup apple cider vinegar
½ cup coconut aminos
¼ cup almond butter
1 tablespoon coconut oil
12 ounces Brussels sprouts, tough ends removed and cut in half
12 ounces carrots (about 4 medium), peeled, ends removed, and cut into 1" chunks
1 cup jasmine rice

1 In a medium bowl, whisk together the broth, lime juice, vinegar, coconut aminos, and almond butter until well combined. Set aside.

2 Press the Sauté button and add the oil to the inner pot. When the oil is melted, add the Brussels sprouts and carrots and sauté, stirring occasionally, 5 minutes. Press the Cancel button.

3 Add the rice and sauce to the inner pot and stir until well combined. Secure the lid.

4 Press the Manual or Pressure Cook button and adjust the time to 3 minutes.

5 When the timer beeps, let pressure release naturally until float valve drops and then unlock lid.

CALORIES: 396 | FAT: 12g | PROTEIN: 10g | SODIUM: 891mg
FIBER: 7g | CARBOHYDRATES: 62g | SUGAR: 7g

Vegan Asian Noodle Bowls

Vegetables and brown rice noodles come together in this vegan version of noodle bowls. Every bit as tasty and satisfying as a version with meat, this recipe takes very minimal prep time and cooks ultrafast in the Instant Pot® pressure cooker. There is nothing better than a warm bowl of noodles and vegetables with a creamy, flavorful sauce.

- **Hands-On Time: 7 minutes**
- **Cook Time: 3 minutes**

Serves 4

½ cup reduced sodium tamari

2 tablespoons rice vinegar

2 tablespoons almond butter

2 tablespoons erythritol

2 cups vegetable broth

2 cups sugar snap peas, roughly chopped

2 large carrots, peeled and thickly sliced (½") on the diagonal

8 ounces uncooked brown rice noodles

¼ cup sliced scallions

4 tablespoons chopped almonds

1 Place the tamari, vinegar, almond butter, erythritol, broth, peas, and carrots in the inner pot and top with the noodles. Secure the lid.

2 Press the Manual or Pressure Cook button and adjust the time to 3 minutes.

3 When the timer beeps, quick-release pressure until float valve drops and then unlock lid.

4 Carefully stir the ingredients. Portion into four bowls and top with scallions and a sprinkle of almonds.

CALORIES: 367 | **FAT**: 9g | **PROTEIN**: 11g | **SODIUM**: 1,152mg
FIBER: 7g | **CARBOHYDRATES**: 67g | **SUGAR**: 7g

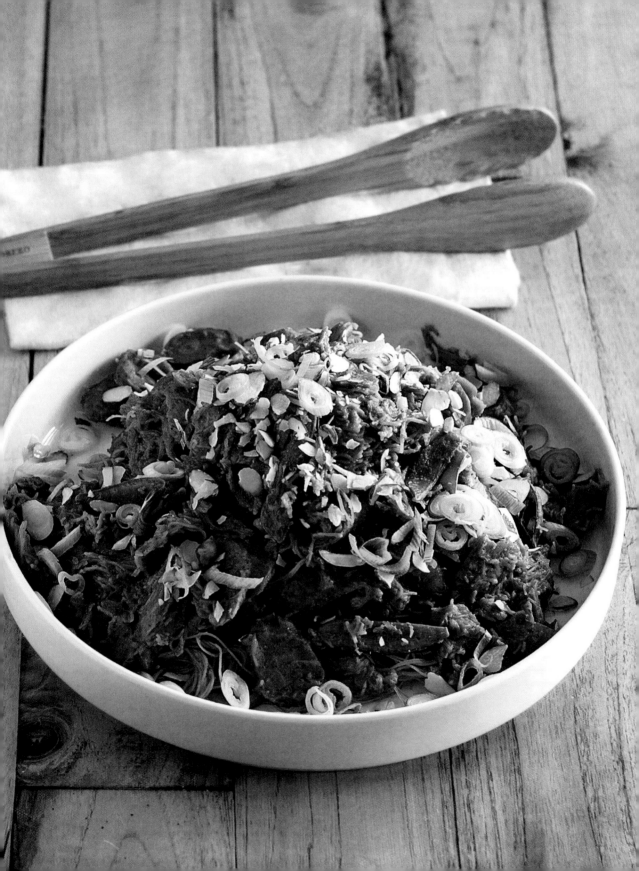

Lentil Muffins

Lentils and vegetables are combined to create meatless muffins that make a wonderful vegetarian main course. Each person gets two individual muffins, and then all you'll need to add is a green salad for a complete meal. To save time, canned lentils can be used for this savory meatless muffin recipe.

- **Hands-On Time: 10 minutes**
- **Cook Time: 17 minutes**

Serves 3

½ tablespoon avocado oil
¼ cup diced onion
⅛ cup diced celery
⅛ cup diced carrots
1 clove garlic, minced
1 large egg
1½ cups cooked lentils
½ tablespoon Italian seasoning blend
1 tablespoon tomato paste
½ tablespoon Dijon mustard
½ cup gluten-free panko bread crumbs
¼ teaspoon salt
⅛ teaspoon black pepper

1 Press the Sauté button and add the oil to the inner pot. Allow the oil to heat 1 minute, and then add the onion, celery, and carrots. Let them cook, stirring frequently, 5 minutes. Add the garlic and sauté an additional 30 seconds. Press the Cancel button.

2 In a large bowl, lightly beat the egg. Add the lentils, Italian seasoning, tomato paste, mustard, bread crumbs, salt, pepper, and the vegetable mixture. Stir until the ingredients are well combined.

3 Place six silicone muffin cups inside a 6" cake pan. Divide the mixture into the six cups. Cover with aluminum foil.

4 Pour 1 cup water into the inner pot, stirring with a wooden spoon to ensure there are no food bits stuck to the pot. Place the steam rack inside and place the cake pan with the lentil muffins on top of the steam rack. Secure the lid.

5 Press the Manual or Pressure Cook button and adjust the time to 10 minutes.

6 When the timer beeps, quick-release pressure until float valve drops and then unlock lid.

7 Carefully remove the pan from the inner pot and remove the aluminum foil. Let the lentil muffins rest 5–10 minutes before serving.

CALORIES: 345 | **FAT**: 8g | **PROTEIN**: 16g | **SODIUM**: 1,521mg
FIBER: 10g | **CARBOHYDRATES**: 48g | **SUGAR**: 3g

Desserts

Sugar is one of the most inflammatory foods out there, so can you actually enjoy desserts when trying to follow an anti-inflammatory diet? The answer is YES!

First, once you are following an anti-inflammatory diet for a period of time and eliminate or reduce the amount of sugar you consume, you'll notice your cravings change. That's when nature's bounty starts to taste delicious. Can fresh fruit actually be a satisfying dessert? Absolutely. Just try the Cinnamon Pineapple and try to argue that it doesn't tantalize your taste buds.

There are times when occasion calls for more than fruit for dessert. Don't worry, this chapter provides options that won't be inflammatory. There are some natural sugar substitutes used in these recipes that won't have the same effects on your body as refined white sugar.

Gluten is also known to be an inflammatory protein, and that's why you won't find any recipes using wheat flour in this book. But how can you make cakes or crisps without the standard wheat flour? Instead of refined white flour, you'll find alternatives like almond flour and coconut flour, which can be used to create comforting desserts that will actually nourish your body as well as satisfy your soul.

Vegan Banana Pudding Cake

If you've never experienced a pudding cake, you're in for a treat. Not quite pudding, not quite cake, this warm Vegan Banana Pudding Cake will leave you dreaming of it long after you polish off your serving. Strong banana flavor is complemented with hints of vanilla and cinnamon, and the chopped pecan topping is simply perfection.

- **Hands-On Time: 10 minutes**
- **Cook Time: 20 minutes**

Serves 6

3 tablespoons ground golden flaxseed meal

10 tablespoons water, divided

1¾ cups mashed banana (about 3 bananas)

¼ cup avocado oil

1 teaspoon pure vanilla extract

2 cups almond flour

½ cup erythritol

1 teaspoon baking powder

¼ teaspoon salt

½ cup chopped pecans

½ teaspoon ground cinnamon

1 In a small bowl, combine the flaxseed and 9 tablespoons water and give it time to gel.

2 In a large bowl, whisk together the flaxseed and water mixture, banana, oil, and vanilla.

3 Add the flour, erythritol, baking powder, and salt and stir to combine well.

4 Spray a 7" cake pan with nonstick cooking spray. Pour the batter into the pan.

5 In a small bowl, combine the chopped pecans, cinnamon, and 1 tablespoon water. Sprinkle on top of the cake batter.

6 Pour 1 cup water into the inner pot and place a steam rack inside. Place the pan on top of the steam rack. Secure the lid.

7 Press the Manual or Pressure Cook button and adjust the time to 20 minutes.

8 When the timer beeps, quick-release pressure until float valve drops and then unlock lid. Spoon into six bowls and serve.

CALORIES: 434 | **FAT**: 35g | **PROTEIN**: 10g | **SODIUM**: 178mg
FIBER: 7g | **CARBOHYDRATES**: 42g | **SUGAR**: 10g

Coconut Cake

Transport yourself to a tropical island with this coconut cake. It's a coconut lover's dream, made with shredded coconut, coconut oil, and coconut milk! Using a springform pan makes it easy to slice and serve this cake, but if you don't have a springform pan a regular 6" cake pan will work also.

- **Hands-On Time: 10 minutes**
- **Cook Time: 40 minutes**

Serves 4

1 cup almond flour
½ cup unsweetened shredded coconut
⅓ cup erythritol
1 teaspoon baking powder
1 teaspoon ground cinnamon
½ teaspoon ground ginger
2 large eggs lightly whisked
¼ cup coconut oil, melted
½ cup unsweetened full-fat canned coconut milk

WHAT IS ERYTHRITOL?

Erythritol is a four-carbon sugar alcohol that occurs naturally in some fruits and fermented foods. Sugar alcohols don't break down in your body, therefore they won't create the same insulin spike that happens when you consume regular sugar. This is why erythritol is a better choice for those following an anti-inflammatory diet.

1 In a large bowl, whisk together the flour, coconut, erythritol, baking powder, cinnamon, and ginger. Add the eggs, coconut oil, and coconut milk and stir until well combined.

2 Spray a 6" springform pan with nonstick cooking spray. Pour the cake batter into the pan.

3 Add 2 cups water to the inner pot and place a steam rack inside. Place the pan on top of the steam rack. Secure the lid.

4 Press the Manual or Pressure Cook button and adjust the time to 40 minutes.

5 When the timer beeps, let pressure release naturally for 10 minutes, then quick-release any remaining pressure until float valve drops, then unlock lid.

6 Allow the cake to cool 5–10 minutes before slicing to serve.

CALORIES: 555 | FAT: 53g | PROTEIN: 10g | SODIUM: 160mg
FIBER: 5g | CARBOHYDRATES: 27g | SUGAR: 2g

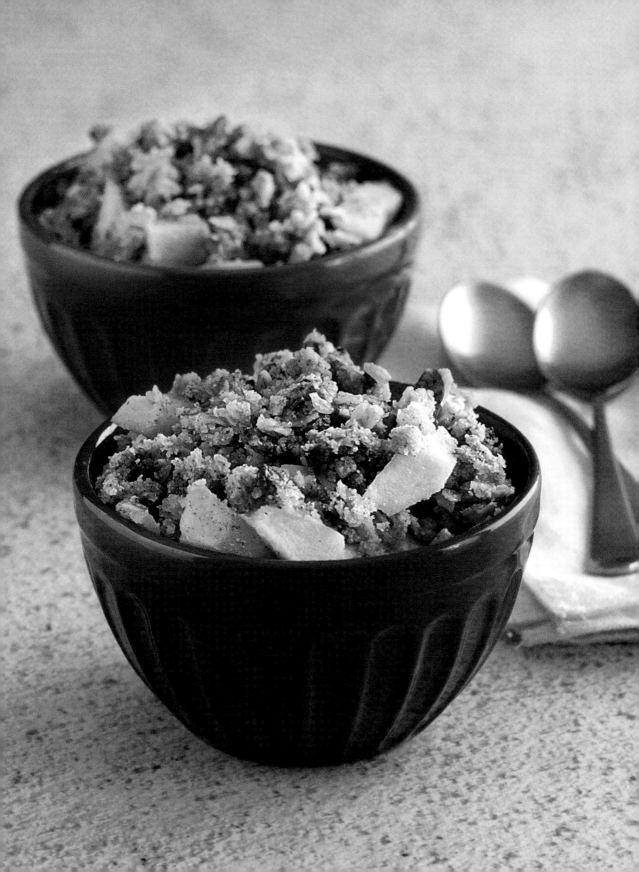

Apple Crisp

Apple Crisp is a staple fall dessert, but it can be enjoyed all year long. With just a few simple swaps, apple crisp becomes a healthier dessert that can help you fight inflammation. Almond flour takes the place of wheat flour and no one will ever know this version has no butter. You can use any kind of apples for this tasty dessert.

- **Hands-On Time: 10 minutes**
- **Cook Time: 17 minutes**

Serves 4

For the Filling

4 large apples, peeled, cored, and cut into wedges

2 tablespoons lemon juice

¼ cup erythritol

¼ teaspoon ground cinnamon

1 teaspoon pure vanilla extract

2 tablespoons almond flour

For the Topping

1 cup almond flour

⅓ cup erythritol

1 cup old fashioned rolled oats

½ cup chopped pecans

¾ teaspoon ground cinnamon

1½ teaspoons vanilla extract

¼ cup coconut oil

2 tablespoons water

1 **To make the Filling:** In a medium bowl, combine the filling ingredients: apples, lemon juice, erythritol, cinnamon, vanilla, and almond flour. Transfer to a 6" cake pan and set aside.

2 **To make the Topping:** In a large bowl, combine the topping ingredients: almond flour, erythritol, oats, pecans, cinnamon, vanilla extract, oil, and water. Use your hands to incorporate the coconut oil into the rest of the ingredients evenly.

3 Pour the topping over the apple filling.

4 Pour 2 cups water into the inner pot and place the steam rack inside. Secure the lid.

5 Press the Manual or Pressure Cook button and adjust the time to 17 minutes.

6 When the timer beeps, quick-release pressure until float valve drops and then unlock lid. Spoon into four bowls and serve.

CALORIES: 600 | **FAT**: 40g | **PROTEIN**: 12g | **SODIUM**: 0mg
FIBER: 10g | **CARBOHYDRATES**: 82g | **SUGAR**: 25g

Blueberry Crisp

Apples shouldn't have all the fun when it comes to the popular dessert known as a crisp. Blueberries are the perfect companion for the vanilla-oat topping, and this time sliced almonds provide a welcome crunch. Orange juice and zest brighten the entire dessert, and with frozen blueberries this is a dessert you can enjoy all year round.

- **Hands-On Time: 10 minutes**
- **Cook Time: 17 minutes**

Serves 4

For the Filling

1 (10-ounce) bag frozen blueberries

2 tablespoons fresh orange juice

¼ cup erythritol

1 teaspoon pure vanilla extract

2 tablespoons almond flour

1 teaspoon orange zest

For the Topping

1 cup almond flour

⅓ cup erythritol

1 cup old fashioned rolled oats

½ cup sliced almonds

1½ teaspoons pure vanilla extract

¼ cup coconut oil

2 tablespoons fresh orange juice

1. **To make the Filling:** In a medium bowl, combine the filling ingredients: the blueberries, orange juice, erythritol, vanilla, flour, and orange zest. Transfer to a 6" cake pan and set aside.

2. **To make the Topping:** In another bowl, combine the topping ingredients: the flour, erythritol, oats, almonds, vanilla, oil, and orange juice. Use your hands to incorporate the oil into the rest of the ingredients evenly.

3. Pour the topping over the blueberry filling.

4. Pour 2 cups water into the inner pot and place the steam rack inside. Place the cake pan on top of the steam rack. Secure the lid.

5. Press the Manual or Pressure Cook button and adjust the time to 17 minutes.

6. When the timer beeps, quick-release pressure until float valve drops and then unlock lid. Spoon into four bowls and serve.

CALORIES: 509 | FAT: 36g | PROTEIN: 13g | SODIUM: 0mg
FIBER: 9g | CARBOHYDRATES: 64g | SUGAR: 9g

Cinnamon Apples

There's not much better than having warm Cinnamon Apples to finish your meal. Experiment with different types of apples, or mix and match for contrasting tart and sweet flavors.

- **Hands-On Time: 10 minutes**
- **Cook Time: 0 minutes**

Serves 4

1 tablespoon coconut oil

5 medium apples, peeled, cored, and cut into large chunks

1½ teaspoons ground cinnamon

1 tablespoon water

1 tablespoon lemon juice

1 Press the Sauté button and put the oil in the inner pot to melt.

2 Once the oil is melted, add the apples, cinnamon, water, and lemon juice and stir to combine. Press the Cancel button. Secure the lid.

3 Press the Manual or Pressure Cook button and adjust the time to 0 minutes.

4 When the timer beeps, quick-release pressure until float valve drops and then unlock lid. Serve warm.

CALORIES: 128 | **FAT**: 3g | **PROTEIN**: 1g | **SODIUM**: 0mg
FIBER: 3g | **CARBOHYDRATES**: 27g | **SUGAR**: 20g

Cinnamon Pineapple

Sometimes dessert doesn't need to be complicated. The simple delight of pineapple cooked in coconut oil and cinnamon will make you realize how flavorful and satisfying fresh fruit can be. The Instant Pot® is the perfect cooking vessel for this simple dessert as it gets the job done quickly and intensifies the pineapple's natural sweetness.

- **Hands-On Time: 10 minutes**
- **Cook Time: 2 minutes**

Serves 6

2 tablespoons coconut oil

1 large pineapple, cored and cut into 2" pieces

1½ teaspoons ground cinnamon

1 Press the Sauté button and add the oil to the inner pot.

2 When the oil is melted, add the pineapple and cinnamon and stir to combine. Press the Cancel button. Secure the lid.

3 Press the Manual or Pressure Cook button and adjust the time to 2 minutes.

4 When the timer beeps, quick-release pressure until float valve drops and then unlock lid.

CALORIES: 115 | **FAT**: 4g | **PROTEIN**: 1g | **SODIUM**: 1mg
FIBER: 2g | **CARBOHYDRATES**: 20g | **SUGAR**: 15g

Banana Chocolate Chip Bundt Cake

Bananas and chocolate are a match made in heaven, and thanks to stevia-sweetened chocolate chips that are readily available today (check online if your supermarket doesn't carry them yet) you can enjoy this combo even on an anti-inflammatory diet. Using a small Bundt cake pan makes a stunning dessert you'll love serving to guests.

- **Hands-On Time: 15 minutes**
- **Cook Time: 55 minutes**

Serves 8

½ cup room temperature coconut oil
1 cup monk fruit sweetener
2 large eggs, room temperature
3 medium bananas, mashed
2 cups oat flour
1½ teaspoons baking soda
½ teaspoon salt
½ cup stevia-sweetened chocolate chips

1 In a large bowl of a stand mixer with a paddle attachment, add the oil, sweetener, and eggs and beat together on medium speed until well combined.

2 Add the mashed banana and beat until combined.

3 Add the flour, baking soda, and salt and beat again until combined.

4 Remove the paddle attachment and stir in the chocolate chips.

5 Spray a 6" Bundt cake pan with cooking oil. Transfer the batter into the pan. Place a paper towel over the top of the pan and then cover with aluminum foil.

6 Add 1½ cups water to the Instant Pot® inner pot and then place a steam rack inside. Place the Bundt pan on the steam rack. Secure the lid.

7 Press the Manual or Pressure Cook button and adjust the time to 55 minutes.

8 When the timer beeps, let pressure release naturally for 10 minutes, then quick-release any remaining pressure until float valve drops, then unlock lid.

9 Allow to cool completely before removing from pan and slicing to serve.

CALORIES: 329 | **FAT**: 21g | **PROTEIN**: 7g | **SODIUM**: 404mg
FIBER: 7g | **CARBOHYDRATES**: 60g | **SUGAR**: 9g

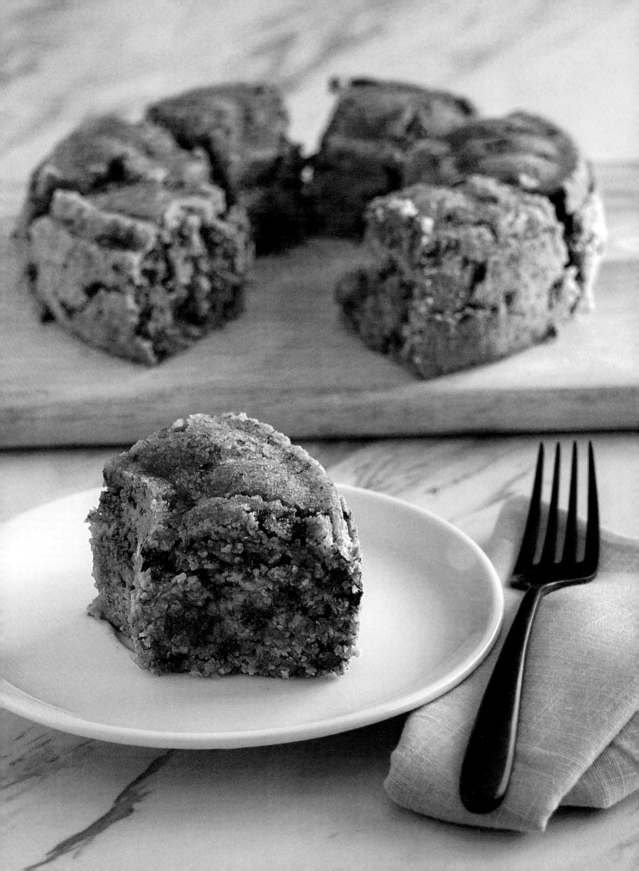

Warm Vegan Caramel Apple Dip

When you mix maple syrup with tahini, you get the most incredibly complex, deep flavors that mimic traditional caramel! This dip is amazing warm, but works well as a cold dip too.

- **Hands-On Time: 5 minutes**
- **Cook Time: 1 minute**

Serves 10

2 cups pitted dates
½ cup tahini
¼ cup maple syrup
¼ cup water, plus more if needed

1 Place the dates, tahini, maple syrup and ¼ cup water in the inner pot of the Instant Pot® and stir to combine. Secure the lid.

2 Press the Manual or Pressure Cook button and adjust the time to 1 minute.

3 When the timer beeps, quick-release pressure until float valve drops and then unlock lid.

4 Allow the mixture to cool slightly, and then transfer to a blender.

5 Blend the mixture on high until super smooth, adding additional water as needed, 1 tablespoon at a time, if the mixture is too thick.

CALORIES: 171 | **FAT**: 6g | **PROTEIN**: 3g | **SODIUM**: 10mg
FIBER: 3g | **CARBOHYDRATES**: 30g | **SUGAR**: 23g

Easiest Vanilla Pumpkin Pudding

Making pudding has never been so easy as when you make it in the Instant Pot®! Flavors of vanilla and pumpkin come together with notes of cinnamon, ginger, nutmeg, and clove for a creamy pudding that's dairy-free and sweetened with pure maple syrup. Maple syrup's deep flavor lends itself well to these classically fall flavors and adds a number of essential minerals.

- **Hands-On Time: 10 minutes**
- **Cook Time: 5 minutes**

Serves 6

1 (13.66-ounce) can unsweetened full-fat coconut milk
1 large egg
½ cup canned pumpkin purée
½ cup pure maple syrup
1 tablespoon pure vanilla extract
2 teaspoons pumpkin pie spice
2 teaspoons arrowroot powder

1 In a medium bowl, whisk together the coconut milk, egg, pumpkin purée, maple syrup, and vanilla until you have a very smooth mixture.

2 Stir in the pumpkin pie spice and arrowroot powder.

3 Transfer the mixture to a 6" cake pan.

4 Pour 2 cups water into the inner pot and place the steam rack inside. Place the cake pan on top of the steam rack. Secure the lid.

5 Press the Manual or Pressure Cook button and adjust the time to 5 minutes.

6 When the timer beeps, let pressure release naturally for 2 minutes, then quick-release any remaining pressure until float valve drops, then unlock lid.

7 Stir the pudding and then transfer it to a glass container with a lid. Chill in the refrigerator 1 hour or more before serving.

CALORIES: 272 | **FAT**: 17g | **PROTEIN**: 7g | **SODIUM**: 70mg
FIBER: 1g | **CARBOHYDRATES**: 23g | **SUGAR**: 17g

Orange Walnut Coffee Cake

Creating gluten-free cakes with different flours can be frustrating because the result is often a dry, crumbly cake. Cakes cooked in the Instant Pot®, however, stay unbelievably moist, even when they're made without wheat flour. This coffee cake, with its orange flavor and crunchy walnut topping, is one you'll want to make over and over!

- **Hands-On Time: 15 minutes**
- **Cook Time: 40 minutes**

Serves 4

3 large eggs

4½ tablespoons pure maple syrup, divided

Zest from 1 medium orange

1 tablespoon fresh orange juice

1 teaspoon pure vanilla extract

1⅓ cups almond flour

1 teaspoon baking powder

¾ teaspoon ground cinnamon, divided

½ teaspoon salt

½ cup walnut pieces

1 In a medium bowl, whisk together the eggs, 4 tablespoons maple syrup, orange zest, orange juice, and vanilla. Add in the flour, baking powder, ½ teaspoon cinnamon, and salt.

2 Transfer the mixture to a 6" cake pan.

3 In a small bowl, mix together the walnuts, ¼ teaspoon cinnamon, and ½ tablespoon maple syrup. Sprinkle on the top of the cake and cover it with aluminum foil.

4 Pour 1 cup water into the inner pot and place a steam rack inside. Place the cake pan on top of the steam rack. Secure the lid.

5 Press the Manual or Pressure Cook button and adjust the time to 40 minutes.

6 When the timer beeps, quick-release pressure until float valve drops and then unlock lid. Allow the cake to cool completely before slicing.

CALORIES: 430 | **FAT**: 31g | **PROTEIN**: 15g | **SODIUM**: 468mg
FIBER: 6g | **CARBOHYDRATES**: 27g | **SUGAR**: 16g

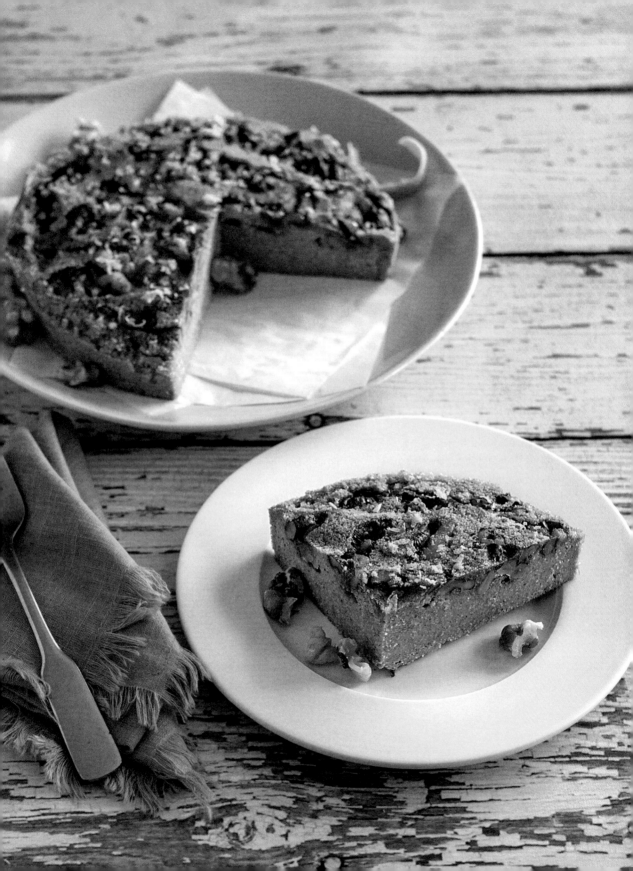

Caramelized Plantains

Plantains resemble bananas, and they are close relatives of bananas, but they are starchier and have less sugar. They are a great source of vitamins A, C, and B$_6$, and also magnesium. When cooking in coconut oil, cinnamon, and maple syrup, they make a simple and delicious dessert that's healthy enough to be eaten as a snack too!

- **Hands-On Time: 5 minutes**
- **Cook Time: 0 minutes**

Serves 4

1 tablespoon coconut oil

3 medium ripe plantains, peeled and sliced thickly on the diagonal

¼ teaspoon salt

1 teaspoon ground cinnamon

2 tablespoons pure maple syrup

¼ cup water

1 Put the oil in the inner pot and press the Sauté button.

2 Once the oil is melted, add the plantains, salt, and cinnamon. Stir until the plantains are coated in the oil and cinnamon. Press the Cancel button.

3 Stir in the maple syrup and water. Secure the lid.

4 Press the Manual or Pressure Cook button and adjust the time to 0 minutes.

5 When the timer beeps, quick-release pressure until float valve drops and then unlock lid.

6 Transfer to bowls for serving.

CALORIES: 220 | **FAT**: 4g | **PROTEIN**: 2g | **SODIUM**: 151mg
FIBER: 3g | **CARBOHYDRATES**: 50g | **SUGAR**: 26g

Blueberry Pudding Cake

While ground flaxseed meal takes the place of eggs in this recipe, making it perfect for anyone with an egg allergy, it also adds some inflammatory-fighting omega-3 fatty acids. It's wonderful when the ingredients that help make a great dessert also nourish your body, and that's the case with this Blueberry Pudding Cake.

- **Hands-On Time: 10 minutes**
- **Cook Time: 20 minutes**

Serves 6

3 tablespoons ground golden flaxseed meal

9 tablespoons water

1¼ cups unsweetened cinnamon applesauce

¼ cup avocado oil

1 teaspoon pure vanilla extract

2¼ cups almond flour, divided

¾ cup erythritol, divided

1 teaspoon baking powder

¼ teaspoon salt

½ cup sliced almonds

½ teaspoon ground cinnamon

1½ cups blueberries

1 In a small bowl, combine the flaxseed and water and give it time to gel.

2 In a large bowl, whisk together the flaxseed and water mixture, applesauce, oil, and vanilla.

3 Add 2 cups flour, ½ cup erythritol, baking powder, and salt and stir to combine well.

4 Spray a 7" cake pan with nonstick cooking spray. Pour the batter into the pan.

5 In a small bowl, combine the almonds, cinnamon, blueberries, remaining ¼ cup flour, and ¼ cup erythritol. Sprinkle mixture on top of the cake batter.

6 Pour 1 cup water into the inner pot and place a steam rack inside. Place the pan on top of the steam rack. Secure the lid.

7 Press the Manual or Pressure Cook button and adjust the time to 20 minutes.

8 When the timer beeps, quick-release pressure until float valve drops and then unlock lid. Spoon into six bowls and serve.

CALORIES: 428 | **FAT**: 35g | **PROTEIN**: 12g | **SODIUM**: 180mg **FIBER**: 8g | **CARBOHYDRATES**: 47g | **SUGAR**: 10g

Maple Pecan Pears

This is a perfect dessert to serve when d'Anjou pears are in peak season, during the winter months. This simple dessert proves, once again, that you don't need a long ingredient list or a dessert to be filled with sugar and refined flour for it to satisfy your sweet tooth.

- **Hands-On Time: 5 minutes**
- **Cook Time: 3 minutes**

Serves 4

2 large ripe but firm d'Anjou pears
1½ tablespoons coconut oil, melted
1 tablespoon pure maple syrup
½ teaspoon ground cinnamon
¼ cup chopped pecans

1 Peel the pears and cut them in half length-wise. Carefully scoop out the core and seeds from each half.

2 Press the Sauté button and add the oil to the inner pot. Once the oil melts, place the pears in the inner pot, cut side down, and cook them until they are starting to get browned, about 2–3 minutes. Press the Cancel button.

3 Carefully transfer the pears to a steamer basket. Add ½ cup water to the inner pot and use a spoon to scrape any brown bits that may be stuck to the bottom of the pot. Place the steam rack inside, and place the steamer basket with the pears on top. Secure the lid.

4 Press the Manual or Pressure Cook button and adjust the time to 0 minutes.

5 When the timer beeps, quick-release pressure until float valve drops and then unlock lid. Carefully transfer the pears to a platter.

6 Remove the water and dry the inner pot. Press Sauté button and add the maple syrup and cinnamon. Stir to combine and heat to warm, about 1 minute. Drizzle the heated maple syrup and cinnamon onto the pears and then sprinkle with chopped pecans and serve.

CALORIES: 173 | **FAT**: 9g | **PROTEIN**: 1g | **SODIUM**: 1mg
FIBER: 4g | **CARBOHYDRATES**: 21g | **SUGAR**: 14g

Strawberry Chocolate Chip Mason Jar Cakes

Why make cakes in Mason jars? Mason jars provide convenient, ready-to-go, portion-controlled servings of this delicious cake. Fresh strawberries burst with flavor and pair perfectly with the stevia-sweetened chocolate chips. This recipe couldn't be simpler to make and is always a hit.

- **Hands-On Time: 5 minutes**
- **Cook Time: 15 minutes**

Serves 4

4 large eggs
2 teaspoons pure vanilla extract
1⅓ cups almond flour
¼ cup erythritol
1 teaspoon baking powder
¼ teaspoon salt
1 cup strawberry chunks
½ cup stevia-sweetened chocolate chips

1 In a medium bowl, whisk the eggs and vanilla. Add the flour, erythritol, baking powder, and salt, and stir to combine. Fold in the strawberries and chocolate chips.

2 Spray four (6-ounce) glass Mason jars with cooking oil. Divide the batter into the jars and cover them with aluminum foil.

3 Pour 1 cup water into the inner pot. Place the steam rack inside and place the Mason jars on the rack. Secure the lid.

4 Press the Manual or Pressure Cook button and adjust the time to 15 minutes.

5 When the timer beeps, quick-release pressure until float valve drops and then unlock lid.

6 Carefully remove the Mason jars from the inner pot and allow to cool before serving.

CALORIES: 402 | FAT: 32g | PROTEIN: 17g | SODIUM: 338mg
FIBER: 13g | CARBOHYDRATES: 42g | SUGAR: 10g

Apple Cinnamon Bundt Cake

Oat flour is a whole grain flour made from the whole oat groat, making oat flour a nutritious flour to use in your desserts. It provides fiber, protein, and iron, making dessert something that adds to your nutrition rather than subtracts from it. The subtle, sweet oat flavor complements the apple cinnamon here perfectly.

- **Hands-On Time: 15 minutes**
- **Cook Time: 55 minutes**

Serves 8

½ cup room temperature coconut oil

1 cup monk fruit sweetener

2 large eggs, room temperature

1 cup unsweetened apple sauce

2 cups oat flour

1½ teaspoons baking soda

1 teaspoon ground cinnamon

½ teaspoon salt

1 large apple, peeled, cored, and diced

MAKE YOUR OWN OAT FLOUR

It is extremely easy to make your own oat flour at home. All you need are some rolled oats and a blender. Once you make a big batch, store it in an airtight glass container so you have it on hand.

1 In a large bowl of a stand mixer with a paddle attachment, beat together the oil, sweetener, and eggs on medium speed until well combined.

2 Add the applesauce and beat until combined.

3 Add the flour, baking soda, cinnamon, and salt and beat again until combined.

4 Remove the paddle attachment and stir in the diced apple.

5 Spray a 6" Bundt cake pan with cooking oil. Transfer the batter into the pan. Place a paper towel over the top of the pan and then cover with aluminum foil.

6 Add 1½ cups water to the Instant Pot® inner pot and then place a steam rack inside. Place the Bundt pan on the steam rack. Secure the lid.

7 Press the Manual or Pressure Cook button and adjust the time to 55 minutes.

8 When the timer beeps, let pressure release naturally for 10 minutes, then quick-release any remaining pressure until float valve drops, then unlock lid.

9 Allow to cool completely before removing from pan and slicing to serve.

CALORIES: 266 | **FAT**: 16g | **PROTEIN**: 6g | **SODIUM**: 404mg
FIBER: 3g | **CARBOHYDRATES**: 48g | **SUGAR**: 6g

Zucchini Cake

Zucchini is the perfect neutral-tasting vegetable to add to desserts and breads. Adding vegetables to your cake is always a great idea! Zucchini adds fiber and vitamin C to your grain-free, sugar-free dessert, and this zucchini cake is so moist and tasty that even young children don't mind the green specks.

- **Hands-On Time: 10 minutes**
- **Cook Time: 40 minutes**

Serves 4

½ cup almond flour
¼ cup coconut flour
⅓ cup erythritol
¼ teaspoon salt
1 teaspoon ground cinnamon
¾ teaspoon baking powder
3 large eggs
¼ cup avocado oil
1 teaspoon pure vanilla extract
½ cup shredded zucchini

1 In a medium bowl, whisk together the almond flour, coconut flour, erythritol, salt, cinnamon, and baking powder.

2 In a separate large bowl, whisk together the eggs, oil, and vanilla.

3 Add the dry ingredients to the wet ingredients and stir to combine. Fold in the zucchini.

4 Transfer the batter to a 6" cake pan and cover with aluminum foil.

5 Pour 1 cup water into the inner pot and add the steam rack inside. Place the cake pan on the rack. Secure the lid.

6 Press the Manual or Pressure Cook button and adjust the time to 40 minutes.

7 When the timer beeps, quick-release pressure until float valve drops and then unlock lid. Allow the cake to cool completely before slicing and serving.

CALORIES: 291 | **FAT**: 24g | **PROTEIN**: 9g | **SODIUM**: 295mg
FIBER: 5g | **CARBOHYDRATES**: 25g | **SUGAR**: 3g

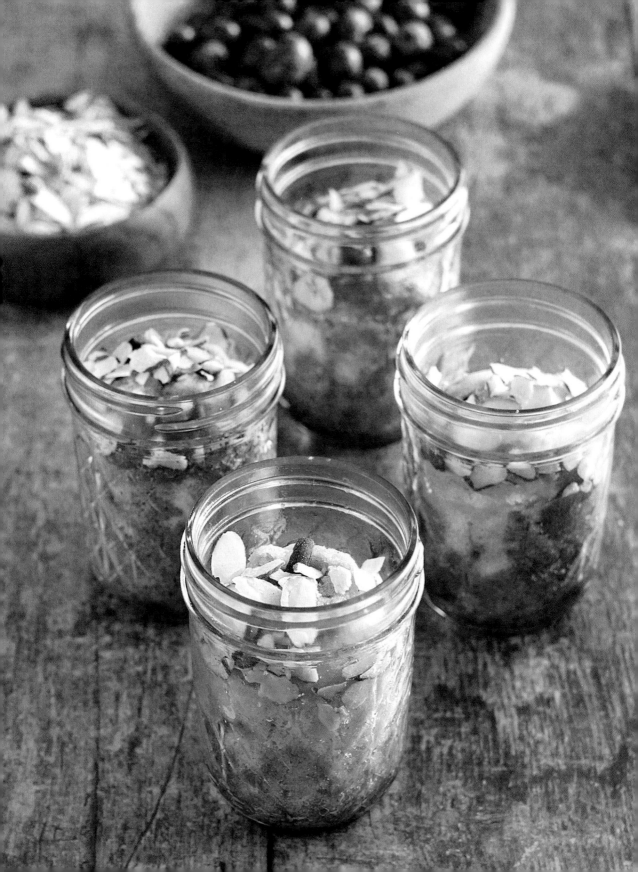

Blueberry Almond Mason Jar Cakes

Blueberries are one of the most antioxidant-filled foods on the planet. Their deep blue color signifies the presence of powerful phytonutrients that help your body reduce damage from free radicals. All of that in a delicious fruit package! Here the blueberries are a juicy addition to these delicious Mason jar cakes.

- **Hands-On Time: 5 minutes**
- **Cook Time: 15 minutes**

Serves 4

4 large eggs

2 teaspoons pure vanilla extract

1⅓ cups almond flour

¼ cup erythritol

1 teaspoon baking powder

¼ teaspoon salt

1 cup blueberries

¼ cup sliced almonds

1 In a medium bowl, whisk the eggs and vanilla. Add the flour, erythritol, baking powder, and salt, and stir to combine. Fold in the blueberries.

2 Spray four (6-ounce) glass Mason jars with cooking oil. Divide the batter into the jars, top each jar with some of the almonds, and cover them with aluminum foil.

3 Pour 1 cup water into the inner pot. Place the steam rack inside and place the Mason jars on the rack. Secure the lid.

4 Press the Manual or Pressure Cook button and adjust the time to 15 minutes.

5 When the timer beeps, quick-release pressure until float valve drops and then unlock lid.

6 Carefully remove the Mason jars from the inner pot and allow to cool before serving.

CALORIES: 345 | **FAT**: 26g | **PROTEIN**: 16g | **SODIUM**: 338mg
FIBER: 6g | **CARBOHYDRATES**: 28g | **SUGAR**: 6g

Coconut Chocolate Rice Pudding

Just when you thought rice pudding couldn't get any better, this recipe uses rich coconut milk and chocolate. This is one dessert that tastes anything but healthy and will make you realize just how delicious it can be to follow an anti-inflammatory diet. No deprivation here!

- **Hands-On Time: 2 minutes**
- **Cook Time: 8 minutes**

Serves 8

1 cup Arborio rice
1½ cups water
¼ teaspoon salt
2 cups unsweetened full-fat canned coconut milk, divided
½ cup erythritol
2 large eggs
½ teaspoon pure vanilla extract
¾ cup stevia-sweetened chocolate chips

WHEN COCONUT MILK SEPARATES

You will often notice that when you open a can of coconut milk, there is a separation of the fat and water. For best results, it's a great idea to mix it back together before using it in any recipe.

1 Add the rice, water, and salt to the inner pot. Secure the lid.

2 Press the Manual or Pressure Cook button and adjust the time to 3 minutes.

3 When the timer beeps, let pressure release naturally for 10 minutes, then quick-release any remaining pressure until float valve drops, then unlock lid.

4 Add 1½ cups coconut milk and erythritol to rice in the inner pot; stir to combine.

5 In a small bowl, whisk eggs with remaining ½ cup coconut milk, and vanilla. Pour through a fine-mesh strainer into the inner pot.

6 Press the Sauté button and cook, stirring constantly until mixture starts to boil, about 5 minutes. Press the Cancel button.

7 Stir in the chocolate chips and spoon into bowls.

CALORIES: 294 | **FAT**: 19g | **PROTEIN**: 6g | **SODIUM**: 97mg
FIBER: 7g | **CARBOHYDRATES**: 47g | **SUGAR**: 5g

Banana Nice Cream Sundae with Strawberry Sauce

Frozen bananas. It's amazing what they can do. Process them in the food processor, and you've got a one-ingredient "nice cream" treat that will surprise you! Topped with a warm strawberry sauce that is made quickly in your Instant Pot®, this is soon to be a favorite healthy dessert.

- **Hands-On Time: 10 minutes**
- **Cook Time: 1 minute**

Serves 6

1 pound strawberries, hulled and chopped
2 tablespoons fresh lemon juice
½ cup erythritol
1 teaspoon arrowroot powder
½ teaspoon water
6 large ripe bananas, sliced and frozen

HOW DO YOU LIKE YOUR ICE CREAM?

Bananas blend to a lovely, creamy treat, but the mixture does melt quickly. Served right away, the blended frozen bananas have the texture of soft-serve ice cream. For a harder texture, freeze the blended bananas in a covered bread pan for a few hours after processing.

1 Add the strawberries, lemon juice, and erythritol to the inner pot. Secure the lid.

2 Press the Manual or Pressure Cook button and adjust the time to 1 minute.

3 In a small bowl, mix the arrowroot powder with water to create a slurry.

4 When the timer beeps, let pressure release naturally for 5 minutes, then quick-release any remaining pressure until float valve drops, then unlock lid.

5 Allow the strawberries to sit 5 minutes, and then stir in the arrowroot slurry and give it a few minutes to thicken.

6 Meanwhile, remove the bananas from the freezer and place them in your food processor. Process the bananas until you have a thick, creamy mixture. Spoon the mixture into six bowls, and spoon some strawberry sauce on the top of each bowl.

CALORIES: 145 | **FAT**: 0g | **PROTEIN**: 2g | **SODIUM**: 2mg
FIBER: 5g | **CARBOHYDRATES**: 53g | **SUGAR**: 20g

US/Metric Conversion Chart

VOLUME CONVERSIONS

US Volume Measure	Metric Equivalent
⅛ teaspoon	0.5 milliliter
¼ teaspoon	1 milliliter
½ teaspoon	2 milliliters
1 teaspoon	5 milliliters
½ tablespoon	7 milliliters
1 tablespoon (3 teaspoons)	15 milliliters
2 tablespoons (1 fluid ounce)	30 milliliters
¼ cup (4 tablespoons)	60 milliliters
⅓ cup	90 milliliters
½ cup (4 fluid ounces)	125 milliliters
⅔ cup	160 milliliters
¾ cup (6 fluid ounces)	180 milliliters
1 cup (16 tablespoons)	250 milliliters
1 pint (2 cups)	500 milliliters
1 quart (4 cups)	1 liter (about)

WEIGHT CONVERSIONS

US Weight Measure	Metric Equivalent
½ ounce	15 grams
1 ounce	30 grams
2 ounces	60 grams
3 ounces	85 grams
¼ pound (4 ounces)	115 grams
½ pound (8 ounces)	225 grams
¾ pound (12 ounces)	340 grams
1 pound (16 ounces)	454 grams

OVEN TEMPERATURE CONVERSIONS

Degrees Fahrenheit	Degrees Celsius
200 degrees F	95 degrees C
250 degrees F	120 degrees C
275 degrees F	135 degrees C
300 degrees F	150 degrees C
325 degrees F	160 degrees C
350 degrees F	180 degrees C
375 degrees F	190 degrees C
400 degrees F	205 degrees C
425 degrees F	220 degrees C
450 degrees F	230 degrees C

BAKING PAN SIZES

American	Metric
8 x 1½ inch round baking pan	20 x 4 cm cake tin
9 x 1½ inch round baking pan	23 x 3.5 cm cake tin
11 x 7 x 1½ inch baking pan	28 x 18 x 4 cm baking tin
13 x 9 x 2 inch baking pan	30 x 20 x 5 cm baking tin
2 quart rectangular baking dish	30 x 20 x 3 cm baking tin
15 x 10 x 2 inch baking pan	30 x 25 x 2 cm baking tin (Swiss roll tin)
9 inch pie plate	22 x 4 or 23 x 4 cm pie plate
7 or 8 inch springform pan	18 or 20 cm springform or loose bottom cake tin
9 x 5 x 3 inch loaf pan	23 x 13 x 7 cm or 2 lb narrow loaf or pâté tin
1½ quart casserole	1.5 liter casserole
2 quart casserole	2 liter casserole

Index

Note: Page numbers in **bold** indicate recipe category lists.

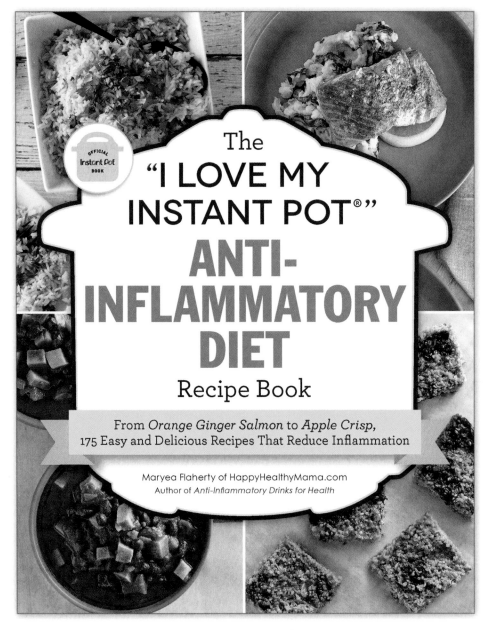
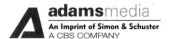